MAYR METHOD DIET FOR BEGINNERS

The complete guide to being healthier, lighter, and with a flat stomach. Including recipes, meal plans, and chewing methods.

Elizabeth Thompson

TABLE OF CONTENTS

INTRODUCTION

The Mayr Method is a diet plan devised in the 1920s by Austrian physician and philosopher Dr. Franz Xaver Mayr. It has garnered notoriety after being credited with helping actor Rebel Wilson lose weight. The program is based on the basis that gut health is critical for weight loss and overall health. It focuses on eliminating particular foods from the diet to improve digestive health and adopt mindful eating techniques such as completely chewing food and avoiding distractions while eating. While the plan is intended to be followed for 14 days and many of the behaviors are intended to develop into long-term habits that promoted overall health. Franz Xaver Mayr founded the F.X. Mayr treatment between 1875 and 1965. After completing his studies in Graz, the medical doctor committed himself totally to the intestines. At the time, he was already convinced that an imbalanced intestinal flora caused a considerable number of ailments. For example, during the First World War, he recognized that protecting the intestines through fasting benefited our organism; since troops who fasted under hardship quickly restored their health. Thus, the Mayr method's primary objective became clear: intestinal rehabilitation. Today, we know for certain that the intestine is the nerve center of our immune system and that a healthy intestine is necessary for optimal health and attractiveness. Often marketed as a fast and quick way to reduce weight, the approach has recently been promoted by celebrities and wellness gurus alike.

While some think the diet is beneficial and simple to follow, others believe it is restrictive and removes key nutritious food groups.

This book examines the Mayr Method in further detail, including what it is, how it works, and whether it is worth doing.

MAYR DIET

THE MAYR METHOD is a well-known diet plan that encourages dieters to maintain healthy habits and make necessary health changes. The Mayr Method diet plan believed that everything is connected to the gut and that what we eat, or do not eat, has an effect on our general health and well-being, including our weight.

The diet was created more than a century ago and entails adopting a mindful eating approach believed to aid weight loss. However, the plan includes rules that, according to two experts, are not sustainable. One expert told Express.co.uk why maintaining a healthy gut is critical; the diet appears quite restrictive.

Jamie Wright, a nutrition expert with Myprotein, stated: "The diet is extremely restrictive and makes several assertions that are supported by scientific evidence." Myprotein's research indicates that the Mayr Method has seen a 150 percent increase in search volume over the last few months.

Despite this, Jame believes that dieting is not necessary to lose weight. "One such claim is the promotion of alkaline foods and the restriction of acidic foods to promote a more desirable PH level in our bodies," he explained.

To summarize, the PH of your food is irrelevant; our bodies regulate PH extremely well, and if they didn't, you'd be quite ill."

According to the expert, the method is intended to cleanse and detoxify the body, which can be quite harmful.

Jamie continued, "A diet will never work for you if it is imposed on your lifestyle." Food is fantastic; I've spent a lot of money and time studying it, so take my word for it when I say I'm a fan. However, we spend an excessive amount of time searching for the next big thing or miracle cure when, in reality, weight loss and sustainable management are quite simple."

Additionally, the diet is governed by many rules.

Nutritionist Jenna Hope explained to Express.co.uk: "The Mayr Method is a restrictive diet with numerous dietary rules, including eating within a set time, avoiding snacking, gluten, and dairy, and abstaining from raw food after 4 p.m."
The method is intended to 'cleanse and detoxify the body,' even though the liver and kidneys' primary function is to remove unwanted toxins from the body.

"Consuming specific foods will not help the body detoxify.

"The rules are intended to promote a significant calorific deficit, which is a critical component of the Mayr Method's weight loss."

Additionally, the expert explained that the weight loss method's rules are "superfluous" to achieve weight loss.
Jenna continued, "Weight loss can be accomplished by following a healthy balanced diet that emphasizes total food intake and portion size." To

lose weight, you must take fewer calories than your body burns.

There are numerous online tools for calculating your calorie deficit, combined with exercise to achieve long-term, healthy weight loss.

Jenna continued, "Stress, sleep deprivation, and other lifestyle factors may also contribute to weight loss."

"In addition, the diet encourages more mindful eating, which benefits appetite regulation, gut health, and micronutrient absorption."

When following the diet, important habits to develop include eating slowly, drinking between meals, and eating a large breakfast and a smaller lunch to promote mindful eating.

However, the nutritionist clarified that "following the Mayr Method is not required to practice mindful eating."

"As an output of the excessive and unnecessary rules, the diet is extremely unsustainable and promotes an unhealthy relationship with food," Jenna continued. As a result, this diet is not suitable for long-term weight loss or maintaining good health.

"This diet is frequently combined with a workout regimen that can also aid in weight loss."

Therefore, if you're attempting to lose weight, you may have heard of the Mayr Method but are unsure whether this weight loss method is safe and effective.

We've discovered a tried-and-true method for helping you lose weight and improve your health while balancing your busy life and assisting your family in living a healthier lifestyle as well.

Nonetheless, there is an awesome deal of information (and misinformation) available, and we want to help educate you on everything.

Understanding the Mayr diet and determining if it is right to help you achieve your health, fitness, and weight loss goals!

If you're looking to lose weight, you've probably heard of the Mayr Method diet, but you're not sure if it's a safe and effective method.

<u>This type of diet for weight loss consists of four critical components:</u>

- ✓ Nutrition and gut health
- ✓ Exercise
- ✓ Medicine
- ✓ Awareness

It is predicated on the belief that typical eating patterns and foods poison people's digestive systems.

The Mayr Method plan combines traditional and complementary medicine to treat any existing health problems and improve mental awareness through exercise and proper nutrition. The creators of the Mayr diet tout the benefits of a flatter stomach, increased energy, and glowing skin.

- ✓ **Nutrition and Gut Health**

  <u>When following the Mayr Method for weight loss, adhere to the following nutritional guidelines:</u>

  - Begin the program with sugar and caffeine.
  - Put an end to snacking
  - Consume fewer dairy products
  - Limit your consumption of gluten-containing foods, such as those made with wheat, barley, or rye.
  - Chew foods more thoroughly for a longer time (chew each bite of food 40-60 times)
  - Consume whole foods that are high in alkalines, such as fruits, vegetables, tofu, nuts, seeds, legumes, and fish.

- Steer clear of highly processed foods
- Maintain a state of mindfulness while eating

The simple truth is that when you follow the Mayr Method diet, you will consume mostly healthy, whole foods and will consume fewer calories overall.

✓ **Exercise**

There is more to the Mayr Method than simply altering your eating habits.

- You'll exercise up to six days a week and eat a well-balanced diet.
- To achieve the best results, combine cardiovascular exercise with resistance training.

✓ **Medicine**

Receiving the appropriate medical care for chronic disease risk factors can significantly reduce your risk of developing a debilitating situation such as diabetes, heart disease, or cancer.

Consult your doctor regularly to ensure that your blood pressure, cholesterol, and triglycerides are properly controlled. Medical treatment may be necessary for addition to making healthy lifestyle changes.

If your doctor prescribes medications for chronic diseases, you may be able to reduce your dosage or even stop taking them entirely as you lose weight.

✓ **Awareness**

Each time you eat, keep your attention on the task at hand to avoid being distracted and consuming an excessive amount of calories.

Distractions such as playing with your phone, watching television, reading, conversing on the phone or with friends are all common.

Effectiveness of Mayr Diet Method

As long as you do not severely restrict calories or foods, the Mayr Method diet can be a safe and effective way to eat.

Here are the keys to the diet:

i. **Consume Alkaline Foods**

   Numerous whole, minimally processed foods, such as fruits, vegetables, legumes, and nuts, are naturally more alkaline, which is why it is the best idea to consume alkaline foods when following the Mayr Method diet.

   However, you are not required to consume only alkaline foods; if you are in good health, your body can regulate pH levels properly on its own.

ii. **Chewing technique and precautions**

   Chewing each bite of food is laborious and time-consuming and is not always feasible.

However, this strategy may assist you in eating more slowly and consuming fewer calories overall, which is beneficial when attempting to reach your target weight.

Guidelines

- Should chew each bite of food at least 40–60 times.
- Eat your bountiful meal first thing in the morning.
- Put down your food as soon as you feel full.
- After 3 p.m., consume only cooked foods.
- Whenever possible, avoid drinking water with meals.
- After 7 p.m., halt eating.

ADVICE ON BREAKFAST, LUNCH, DINNER, AND SNACK TIMES

Snacks

Avoiding snacks can help you reduce your overall calorie intake for weight loss, as long as you do not overeat at mealtime. Snacks every four to six hours are recommended, as are snacks in between (for example, snack at 10 to 10:30). Additionally, if you are hungry during the day, you should never feel obligated to eat, regardless of how many meals or snacks you have already consumed.

However, you do not have to forego snacks entirely to lose weight effectively.

Indeed, in some cases, skipping snacks can result in in-between-meal fatigue or overeating at mealtime.

Consume a small meal or snack approximately every few hours. Snacking is prohibited, dairy and gluten consumption is restricted, raw foods are avoided after 4 p.m., and breakfast is emphasized with the option of skipping it.

Breakfast

Breakfast promotes good health by improving memory and concentration, lowering "bad" LDL cholesterol levels, and decreasing the risk of creating diabetes, heart disease, and obesity.

It's unclear, however, whether breakfast promotes these healthy habits or whether those who eat it live healthier lifestyles. However, one thing is certain: skipping breakfast can throw off your body's fasting and eating rhythms. When you awaken, your blood sugar level is typically low, which is necessary for your muscles and brain to function optimally. Breakfast contributes to its replenishment. It will assist you in calorie burning throughout the day. Additionally, it provides the energy necessary to accomplish tasks and aids in concentration at work or school. That is just a sampling of the reasons why breakfast is the most important meal of the day.

However, it stated and believed that following the Mayr Method, which focuses on portion control, gut health, inflammation reduction, and the elimination of processed foods, assists in staying in shape. Additionally, mindful eating eliminates snacking, limits dairy and gluten intake, and places a premium on chewing food slowly.

According to an accurate report, the day's largest meal is breakfast, followed by a smaller meal at lunch and a smaller meal at supper. After 3 p.m., raw foods are not recommended. As a result, you should probably eat a substantial breakfast – think organic eggs, spinach, and homemade bread. Additionally, good housekeeping revealed a list of foods permitted on the Mayr plan, including apricots, apples, and berries. Ground oats are permitted, which is ideal for someone who is a big fan of porridge.

Lunch

Lunches, like all meals, should be nutritious and enjoyable. A simple way to contribute to a balanced lunch includes foods from at least three food groups (vegetables, fruits, grains, protein, and dairy/calcium-rich). However, improper lunch regulation may result in the body gaining weight. Meals on the Mayr plan are frequently centered on fish such as salmon or chicken breast, and the star strives to maintain an overall healthy balance of foods. "That is not to say that every week is a healthy week." Certain weeks are simply non-starters, and there is nothing you can do about it." The Mayr plan allows for trout and smoked salmon and skinless turkey breast and tofu when it comes to foods. There are numerous vegetables to choose from, including carrots, potatoes, tomatoes, lettuce, broccoli, and turnips. Certain carbs, such as risotto rice and polenta, make the cut.

Dinner

We envision dinner ingredients to be similar to lunch ingredients, but in a smaller portion – lean protein and plenty of fresh vegetables. Of course, even celebrities have cheating days. Bear in mind that you must continue to treat yourself (albeit only once or twice a week with food). A well-balanced meal plan recommends green tea, water, and pomegranate juice as beverages. Indeed, it sounds quite healthy!

The Mayr plan's new diet entails abstaining from sugar and junk food. However, most days, consuming 3,000 calories and most of them being carbs, one can still feel hungry.

HOW TO IMPROVE DIGESTION BASED ON THE MAYR DIET PLAN

Everybody occasionally experiences digestive symptoms such as indigestion, gas, heartburn, nausea, constipation, or diarrhea.
When these symptoms occur frequently, they can significantly disrupt your life.

Fortunately, diet and lifestyle changes can improve gut health. The Mayr Diet plan and method are based on natural ways to improve your digestion. The following evidence supports the Mayr Diet plan and method for improving digestion:

Consume Real Food

The diet, which is high in refined carbohydrates, saturated fat, and food additives, has been associated with an increased risk of developing digestive disorders.
Meals additives, such as glucose, salt, and other chemicals, have been implicated in promoting gut inflammation, resulting in a condition known as

leaky gut. Trans fats are present in a wide variety of processed foods. They are well-known for their detrimental effects on cardiovascular health, but they have also been linked to an increased risk of developing ulcerative colitis, an inflammatory bowel disease.

Additionally, processed foods such as low-calorie beverages and ice creams frequently contain artificial sweeteners, which have been linked to digestive problems.

According to one study, consuming 50 grams of the artificial sweetener xylitol caused 70% of people to experience bloating and diarrhea, while 75 grams of the sweetener erythritol caused 60% of people to experience the same symptoms.

Additionally, studies indicate that artificial sweeteners may increase the number of harmful gut bacteria in your body.

Unbalanced gut bacteria have been associated with irritable bowel syndrome (IBS) and irritable bowel diseases such as ulcerative colitis and Crohn's disease.

Fortunately, scientific evidence suggests that nutrient-dense diets may help prevent digestive diseases.

Consequently, consuming a diet rich in whole foods and avoiding processed foods may be the best option for optimal digestion.

Consume an Adequate Amount of Fiber

It is widely accepted that fiber is beneficial for digestion.

Soluble fiber absorbs water and assists your stool in retaining its bulk. Insoluble fiber acts as a giant toothbrush, assisting your digestive tract in maintaining proper function.

Soluble fiber is detected in oat bran, legumes, nuts, and seeds, while insoluble fiber is found in vegetables, whole grains, and wheat bran.

A high-fiber diet has been associated with a decreased risk of developing digestive conditions such as ulcers, reflux, hemorrhoids, diverticulitis, and irritable bowel syndrome.

Prebiotics are another type of fiber that supports the growth of beneficial bacteria in the gut. Consuming a diet high in this fiber has been shown to reduce the risk of developing inflammatory bowel disease. Numerous fruits, vegetables, and grains contain prebiotics.

Increase Your Consumption of Healthy Fats

Sufficient fat consumption may be necessary for proper digestion. Fat satisfies you after a meal and is frequently required for proper nutrient absorption.

Omega-3 fatty acids have also been appeared to lower the risk of developing inflammatory bowel diseases like ulcerative colitis.

Flaxseeds, chia seeds, nuts (especially walnuts), and fatty fish such as salmon, mackerel, and sardines are high in beneficial omega-3 fatty acids.

Maintain proper hydration

Inadequate fluid consumption is a frequent cause of constipation.

Experts recommend drinking 50–66 ounces (1.5–2 liters) of non-caffeinated fluids daily to avoid constipation. Living in a hot climate or engage in strenuous exercise, you may need more.

In support of water, herbal teas and other non-caffeinated beverages such as seltzer water can help you meet your fluid requirements.

Another way to meet your fluid requirements is to consume water-dense fruits and vegetables such as melons, strawberries, grapefruit, cucumber, zucchini, celery, tomatoes, and peaches.

Take Control of Your Stress

Stress can hurt your digestive system. It has been connected to stomach ulcers, diarrhea, constipation, and irritable bowel syndrome.

Stress hormones have a crucial impact on digestion. When you're in fight-or-flight mode, your body believes there's no time for rest or digestion. Stress causes blood and energy to be diverted away from the digestive system.

Additionally, the gut and the brain are inextricably linked — whatever affects the brain may also affect digestion.
Irritable bowel syndrome symptoms are improved by stress management, meditation, and relaxation training. Additionally, cognitive behavioral therapy, acupuncture, and yoga have been shown to improve digestive symptoms.

As a result, incorporating stress management techniques such as deep belly breathing, meditation, or yoga may be turned to one's advantage to both your mental and physical health.

Consume Consciously

If you're not paying attention, it's easy to eat too much too quickly, which can result in bloating, gas, and indigestion.

The practice of mindful eating entails paying attention to all aspects of your food and eating process.

Mindfulness can help people with ulcerative colitis, and irritable bowel syndrome (IBS) manage their digestive symptoms.

To consume food mindfully:

- Consume slowly.
- Dedicate your attention to your food by turning off the television and putting away your phone.
- Take note of the appearance and smell of the food on your plate.
- Select each bite of food consciously.
- Be focus on your food's texture, temperature, and flavor.

Masticate Your Food

The digestive process begins in the mouth. Your teeth break down a meal into smaller pieces, allowing the enzymes in your digestive tract to break it down more effectively.

Inadequate chewing has been associated with reduced nutrient absorption.

When you chew your food thoroughly, it takes less effort for your stomach to convert the solid food into the liquid mixture that enters your small intestine.

Saliva is produced when you chew, and the longer you chew, the more saliva is produced. Saliva aids in the breakdown of some of the carbohydrates and fats in your meal, which helps start the mouth's digestive process.

Saliva acts as a fluid in the stomach, mixing with solid food to ensure that it passes easily into the intestines.

By thoroughly chewing your meal, you ensure that you have an adequate supply of saliva for digestion. It may help prevent symptoms such as heartburn and indigestion.

Additionally, chewing has been shown to reduce stress, which may help with digestion.

Get Yourself Moving

Exercise regularly is one of the most effective ways to improve your digestion.

Exercise and gravity aid in the passage of food through the digestive system. As a result, taking a walk following a meal may help your body move things along.

One study found that moderate exercise, such as cycling and jogging, increased gut transit time by nearly 30% in healthy individuals.

Another study found that a daily exercise regimen involving 30 minutes of walking significantly improved symptoms in people with chronic constipation.

Additionally, studies indicate that exercise may help alleviate symptoms of inflammatory bowel diseases through its anti-inflammatory effects, which include a decrease in inflammatory compounds in the body.

Take a Deep Breath and Listen to Your Body

When you wave your hunger and fullness cues, it's easy to overeat, resulting in gas, bloating, and indigestion.
It is a widely held belief that it takes your brain 20 minutes to register that your stomach is full.

While little science supports this claim, it takes time to reach your brain for hormones released by your stomach in response to diet.

Thus, eating slowly and paying attention to how full you are is one way to avoid common digestive problems.
Additionally, emotional eating has a detrimental effect on digestion. According to one study, individuals who ate while anxious experienced increased levels of indigestion and bloating.

Allowing yourself time to unwind before a meal may help alleviate digestive symptoms.

Eliminate Bad Habits

You are aware that unhealthy habits such as smoking, excessive alcohol consumption, and eating late at night are detrimental to your overall health.

Indeed, they may also be to blame for several common digestive problems.

- ✓ Smoking

  The risk of developing acid reflux is nearly doubled when a person smokes.

  Additionally, studies have shown that cessation of smoking alleviates these symptoms.

  Additionally, this unhealthy habit has been linked to stomach ulcers, increased surgical procedures in patients with ulcerative colitis, and gastrointestinal cancers.

If you have digestive issues and smoking cigarettes, consider quitting.

✓ Alcohol

Alcohol can cause your stomach to produce more acid, resulting in heartburn, acid reflux, and stomach ulcers.

Excessive alcohol consumption has been associated with gastrointestinal bleeding.

Additionally, alcohol has been linked to inflammatory bowel diseases, leaky gut syndrome, and harmful changes in gut bacteria.

Reduce your alcohol consumption to aid digestion.

✓ Consumption of Food Late at Night

Consuming food late at night and then sleeping can result in heartburn and indigestion.

Your body requires time to digest, and gravity assists in moving the food you eat in the proper direction.

Additionally, when you lie down, your stomach contents may rise to the surface, causing heartburn. After eating, lying down strongly correlates with an increase in reflux symptoms.

If you have digestive problems at night, wait three to four hours after eating to allow the food to pass from your stomach to your small intestine.

Supplement with Gut-Supporting Nutrients

Certain nutrients may aid in the maintenance of your digestive tract.

✓ Probiotics

Probiotics are beneficial bacteria that, when taken as supplements, may help improve digestive health.

These beneficial bacteria aid in digestion by degrading indigestible fibers that can result in gas and bloating.

Studies have shown that probiotics enhance bloating, gas, and pain symptoms in people with irritable bowel syndrome (IBS).
Additionally, they may alleviate constipation and diarrhea symptoms.
Probiotics are discovered in fermented foods like sauerkraut, kimchi, miso, and live and active cultures in yogurt.
Additionally, they are available in capsule form. A good multi-strain probiotic supplement will contain Lactobacillus and Bifidobacterium strains.

✓ Glutamine

An amino acid that aids in the health of the gut is regarded as Glutamine. It has been shown to decrease intestinal permeability (leaky gut) in critically ill patients (46Trusted Source).

Consume foods such as turkey, soybeans, eggs, and almonds to boost your glutamine levels.

Glutamine can also be taken as a supplement, but consult your healthcare practitioner first to ensure that this is a treatment strategy that is appropriate for you.

✓ Zinc

Zinc is a critical mineral for maintaining a healthy gut, and a deficiency can result in various gastrointestinal disorders.

Zinc supplementation has been demonstrated to be beneficial in treating diarrhea, colitis, leaky gut, and other digestive problems.
Zinc's recommended daily intake (RDI) for women is 8 mg and for men is 11 mg.
Shellfish, beef, and sunflower seeds are all high in zinc.

INFORMATION ON HOW TO DO STOMACH MASSAGE

Abdominal massage, also known as stomach massage, is a gentle, non-invasive treatment that can relax and heal. It's used to cure a wide range of health problems, particularly those involving the stomach, such as bloating, constipation, and digestion problems.

You can do the abdominal massage yourself or schedule an appointment with a massage therapist. After only five(5) or ten(10) minutes of massage per day, you may notice the benefits of abdominal massage. If you are pregnant or not health-wise, consult your doctor before getting an abdominal massage.

How to self-massage your abdomen for bloating and constipation

Abdominal massage comes in a variety of forms. Allowing for basic home use of the technique, we believe anyone performing these techniques at home must have a thorough knowledge of the anatomical regions they can influence with this and other techniques. It's also crucial to recognize whether you're suffering from a type of constipation or bloating that responds to self-massage. Before seeking how to do self abdominal massage, it is always a good idea to seek advice.

While there are many different types of abdominal massage, we prefer to use techniques based on sound anatomical principles and structures within the abdominal cavity. As with most abdominal massage techniques, there are a few things to keep in mind that could affect the technique's success and your ability to learn self-abdominal massage techniques.

If you know you have one of the following conditions, you should avoid self-abdominal massage because it may harm your health. Some of the conditions listed here are absolute reasons you should not self-abdominal, while others are reasons you should seek medical advice before the self-abdominal massage.

Contra-indications, cautions, and modifications of self-abdominal massage

At times, abdominal self-massage may be inappropriate or even contraindicated, and all techniques may require modification. It is suggested that you go and see your practitioner if you have any concerns about any of these possible conditions.

- In the immediate aftermath of abdominal surgery
- Presenting with an active infection or cancer in the pelvic area while undergoing chemotherapy
- Infections that are active and acute
- Abdominal aneurysm
- Diastasis of the rectus femoris
- Diverticular disease that is inflamed
- Blockage or suspicion of blockage of the stomach region
- Possible appendicitis

- The presence of an IUD (intrauterine device for contraception)
- Necessary in the case of uterine prolapse (remove before your session)
- Any serious health problem that concerns you

The optimal technique for self-abdominal massage instruction

The technique described here for self abdominal massage is a simple technique for reducing one's own bloating and feeling a little lighter and freer in one's stomach and digestive system.

Relying on your back while your knees are bent and a pillow or rolled-up towel under your knees if possible. It is primarily to ensure that the muscles in the stomach area are relaxed and less resistant to the massage techniques. The position will make it significantly easier to move one's digestive system and allow for a more fluid movement during the self-abdominal massage. It is critical for the technique to be effective, as the digestive system operates in a highly rhythmic manner known as peristalsis. It enables you to work with, rather than against, the digestive system, thereby encouraging the return of normal function. Additionally, one may choose to work through their clothing, as this may be more convenient at times when direct contact with the skin and abdominal wall is not possible. By slightly raising one's head, one can also assist in relaxing the anterior abdominal wall and upper chest region, which may affect the technique's outcome.

To replicate the flow in one's digestive system, the direction of movement in one's hands must be clockwise (once the stomach has been cleared by working lightly in the opposite direction (anti-clockwise), this helps to unblock the stomach before working in a clockwise direction). The large intestine region is the easier of the two to work on. By improving digestion flow through the large intestine, one can significantly improve bloating and digestive pain symptoms. It indirectly affects the stomach and small intestines because it reduces the backlog in the large intestines, thereby improving the overall transit time in the small and large intestines.

Some critical landmarks to remember when learning how to self-massage the abdomen

Before studying how to do self abdominal massage and performing abdominal self-massage, it is necessary to understand a few lower stomach region landmarks. It will assist you in determining where to begin, end treatments, and the direction in which to move around the stomach. Generally, the pressure depth is between 1 and 2 cm. It enables you to apply sufficient pressure to the stomach/colon to stimulate the digestive system to begin moving. In general, applying more pressure than this may result in abdominal pain or discomfort. If you experience any pain or inconvenience, stop and consult an abdominal massage specialist for assistance or advice with these techniques or gain a thorough understanding of any stomach conditions affecting you before studying how to do self abdominal massage.

If you divide the abdominal region into nine equal boxes, you can visualize the major regions of the stomach and, more importantly, the area in which you will be working. These boxes are frequently referred to as nine quadrants, each of which contains specific organs that you should be aware of if performing this self-abdominal massage technique without guidance.

Other boxes are defined by the lower ribs and diaphragm region when looking at your stomach. These three quadrants contain the organs responsible for the early stages of digestion and the immune system. The upper right quadrant contains the spleen and splenic flexure of the descending colon; should exercise caution in this region if any discomfort or swelling is present, as it may indicate underlying pathology. The liver, gallbladder, and ascending colon's hepatic flexure are located in the upper left quadrant. These are critical landmarks for abdominal self-massage. The transverse colon, the stomach portion of the liver, the duodenum, and the esophagus are located in the central quadrant above the umbilical area but below the ribs. It is particularly sweet because it may be associated with sliding or rolling Hiatus Hernia and may manifest as bloating or digestive discomfort.

Additionally, this region may be affected by duodenal or gastric ulcers, gastritis, or other conditions affecting the stomach, esophagus, duodenum, and occasionally the liver. These upper quadrants are referred to anatomically about the adjacent regions. The epigastric region is the central quadrant. As a result, the left and right quadrants are frequently referred to as the left and right hypochondriac regions, respectively.

As you descend into the next three quadrants, the contents become more condensed, making it easier to discover which organs may be involved if there is any pain in these areas. Left lumbar, umbilical, and right lumbar regions are designated from left to right. The descending colon is located in the left lumbar region, the umbilical region contains mostly small intestines, and the ascending colon is located in the right lumbar region.

The left and right Iliac regions, which lie beneath the left and right lumbar regions, contain digestive organs. The central quadrants define the hypogastric region in the lower part of the stomach. This region may contain small intestines but primarily begins to contain more pelvic organs. In women, the upper part of the uterus may occasionally be palpable here, as well as a distended bladder.

The benefits of abdominal massage

About the American Massage Therapy Association (AMTA), massage therapy can benefit a person's physical, mental, and social well-being. It is believed to benefit overall health and wellness. May obtain additional benefits through abdominal massage.

- **Relieve constipation**

  Massage of the abdomen may aid in the relaxation of the stomach muscles. This, in turn, aids digestion and alleviates constipation.

  A small study investigated the effects of abdominal massage on postoperative constipation. The researchers discovered that people who received abdominal massage — as opposed to a control group that did not receive massage — had the following characteristics:

- ✓ Alleviation of constipation symptoms
- ✓ Increased frequency of bowel movements
- ✓ Shorter intervals between bowel movements

- **Enhance digestion**

abdominal massage's effect on the digestive problems of people who had an endotracheal tube. Individuals who received a 15-minute abdominal massage twice daily for three days improved their symptoms significantly more than those who received no treatment. Additionally, the massage group had less stomach liquid and significantly reduced their abdominal circumference and constipation.

Additional research is required, both in hospital settings and among non-hospitalized individuals.

- **Reduce bloating**

Found the abdominal massage to treat several symptoms associated with excess fluid accumulation in the abdominal cavity (common in cancer patients).

In this study, participants who received a 15-minute abdominal massage twice daily for three days reported experiencing less abdominal bloating. Depression, anxiety, and general well-being all improved as well.

Massage to the abdomen did not affect their other symptoms, including pain, nausea, and fatigue.

- **Additional benefits**

Additionally to the benefits listed previously, abdominal massage Additionally to the benefits listed previously, abdominal massage may:

- ✓ Aid in weight loss
- ✓ Promote relaxation
- ✓ Abdominal muscles are toned and strengthened
- ✓ assist in the release of physical and emotional tension
- ✓ alleviate spasms of the muscles
- ✓ augmentation of blood flow to the abdomen

✓ beneficial to the abdominal organs

TIPS AND A MEAL PLAN FOR FULL-TIME EMPLOYEES

You're on a conference call and have inadvertently found yourself in the kitchen. Before you know it, you're snacking on crackers and dry cereal straight from the box. Or perhaps you became so absorbed in a project that you realized you hadn't eaten anything all day. Perhaps the mentality of "I'll just have a handful of chips while I work" evolved into accidentally eating the entire bag.

Maintaining a healthy diet can not be easy when your home serves as your office. You feel at ease, and there is an abundance of food available. And, unlike at the office, you are free to graze all day and have complete access to the refrigerator. However, these characters can wreak havoc on your waistline, sabotage your weight loss efforts, and put a halt to your productivity.

- **Avoid working in (or close to) the kitchen.**
  Attempt to locate your desk away from the kitchen. If the refrigerator is repeatedly in your line of vision, you may be tempted to wander over and check it (for the tenth time). Decide that you will only enter your kitchen during the workday to prepare a planned snack or meal. (More on this later!) If you're having trouble sticking to this, put a reminder on your refrigerator and pantry that the kitchen is shut until the next meal or snack.

- **Establish a schedule for snacking and meals.**

  Just as you schedule and plan the rest of your day (wake up, workout, shower), schedule and plan when you're going to eat throughout the day. If you know you prefer to eat lunch around noon, schedule accordingly. And, if you enjoy a late afternoon snack, plan for that as well. Consider food in the same way that you would in the office. You cannot graze all day while you are there – so act similarly at home.

- **Ensure that you consume food.**

  Once you're up and running, er, working, it can be difficult to take a break to eat. However, it is critical to recognize your hunger signals and understand that not eating can impair your alertness and productivity. Additionally, eating throughout the day can keep you from becoming a huge hangry mess when 5 p.m. rolls around. Set the alarm on your phone, if possible, to remind you to get up and eat something.

- **Prepare your lunches in advance.**
  Having the freedom to prepare whatever you want for lunch is a liberating experience (and It's a huge plus not to have to stand in line for the work microwave.). However, for some, the freedom is excessive, particularly when it comes to weekday lunches. If possible, meal prep your lunches in advance, just as you would on days when you physically report to work. It also does not have to be anything extravagant. A bag of lettuce, precut vegetables, grilled chicken, and nuts is a straightforward method of meal preparation that eliminates all guesswork. Or perhaps you've resolved to make a veggie omelet for lunch every day. Prepare the vegetables ahead of time to ascertain a quick and healthy lunch.

- **Concentrate on real food.**

We are more productive when we eat a balanced, nutritious diet. It keeps us fuller for longer and aids in concentration. Recognize that what you eat affects your mood and energy level. Consider this the next time you're hungry and tempted to reach for a handful of chocolate in the pantry. Protein, fiber, healthy fats, fruits, and vegetables should all be prioritized. Preparing a menu in advance will help you avoid snacking on whatever looks the tastiest and quickest at the moment.

- **Drink plenty of water.**

  Dehydration can result in headaches and fatigue, both of which are detrimental to productivity. Similarly to how you would fill a water bottle at work to keep at your desk, keep water near your work station at home. If you have water readily available, you're more likely to drink it, which will help you meet your daily water goal of at least 64 ounces. (And PLEASE avoid sugary sodas and juices, which can result in a crash later.)

- **Avoid excessive caffeine.**

  While having unlimited cups of coffee may seem like a great idea, caution should be exercised when it comes to caffeine. Too much is known to let you have headaches, anxiety, digestive problems, and even fatigue – none of which are desirable in any circumstance, but especially not when attempting to work. Limit yourself to two cups of coffee per day to avoid the jittery feeling, and stay away from flavored creamers and other high-calorie additives!

- **Avoid purchasing junk food.**

  Do not stock your refrigerator or pantry in the manner of a vending machine. It may lead to eating just for the sake of eating! Keep junk food as far away from your home as possible, especially foods that you know will cause you to binge. It is said that what is out of sight is out of mind.

- **When you eat, eat simply.**

Now that your coworkers are gone, you might be tempted to work through your lunch break. However, refrain from doing so! Distracted eating can result in overeating and a decrease in satiety (satisfaction and fullness) following the meal. Better still, take a break from work, sit at a table, and enjoy your lunch for a few minutes. You'll get more enjoyment out of the meal, and it may even help you feel more prepared for the remainder of your workday.

- **Before eating, portion out snacks and meals.**

  Do not consume out of the bag or original container because it is much more difficult to keep track of portion sizes. Refer to the serving size indicated on the container if you need more information. Consider the healthy plate method for meals: Half of a 9-inch plate should be made up of non-starchy vegetables, one-fourth should be made up of lean protein (poultry, seafood, beans, eggs, tofu, cottage cheese, or Greek yogurt), and one-fourth should be made up of a high-fiber carbohydrate (fruit, whole grains or starchy vegetables).

MAJOR HEALTH BENEFITS OF FOLLOWING MAYR DIET

Mayr Diet Healthy eating also entails substituting more nutritious foods for those that contain trans fats, added salt, and sugar.
Consuming a nutritious mayr diet has several health benefits, including strengthening bones, protecting the heart, preventing disease, and enhancing mood. The benefits of a nutritious diet, as well as the evidence for them.

1. Heart health

Regarding the Centers for Disease Control and Prevention (CDC), heart disease is the leading cause of death for adults in the United States, according to the Centers for Disease Control and Prevention (CDC).
Adults are evaluated to have some form of cardiovascular disease.

Hypertension, or high blood pressure, is a growing concern. The condition is associated with an increased risk of heart attack, heart failure, and stroke.

According to some sources, lifestyle changes such as increased physical activity and healthy eating can prevent up to 80% of premature heart disease and stroke diagnoses.

Consumption of certain foods can help people lower their blood pressure and maintain a healthy heart.

<u>The mayr diet program makes the following recommendations:</u>

- ✓ Consuming a sufficient amount of vegetables, fruits, and whole grains
- ✓ Selecting low-fat or fat-free dairy products, fish, poultry, beans, nuts, and vegetable oils
- ✓ Limiting consumption of saturated and trans fats, which include fatty meats and full-fat dairy products.
- ✓ Limiting sugar-sweetened beverages and foods
- ✓ Limiting sodium intake to less than 2,300 milligrams per day — ideally, 1,500 milligrams

per day — and increasing potassium, magnesium, and calcium consumption

Fiber-rich foods are also critical for heart health.

The mayr diet's fiber content contributes to improved blood cholesterol levels and reduces the risk of heart disease, stroke, obesity, and type 2 diabetes.

Trans fats have long been associated with heart-related illnesses such as coronary heart disease.

Restriction of certain types of fats can also benefit heart health. Eliminating trans fats, for example, lowers low-density lipoprotein cholesterol levels. This type of cholesterol contributes to plaque accumulation in the arteries, increasing heart attack and stroke risk.

Blood pressure control may also benefit heart health. This can be accomplished by restricting one's daily salt intake to no more than 1,500 milligrams.

Many processed and fast foods contain salt, and anyone wishing to lower their blood pressure should avoid these products.

2. Enhanced gut health

The colon is densely packed with naturally occurring bacteria that are critical for metabolism and digestion.

Additionally, certain strains of bacteria produce vitamins K and B, which are beneficial for the colon. Additionally, these strains aid in the fight against pathogenic bacteria and viruses.

A low-fiber, high-sugar, and high-fat diet alters the gut microbiome, resulting in increased inflammation in the area.

A diet high in vegetables, fruits, legumes, and whole grains, on the other hand, provides a combination of prebiotics and probiotics that promote the growth of beneficial bacteria in the colon.

Probiotics are abundant in these fermented foods:

- Yogurt
- Kimchi
- Sauerkraut
- Miso

- Kefir

Fiber is a readily available prebiotic found in large amounts in legumes, grains, fruits, and vegetables. Additionally, it encourages regular bowel movements, which may aid in the prevention of bowel cancer and diverticulitis.

3. Loss of weight

Maintaining a healthy weight can assist reduce your risk of developing chronic health problems. Obesity and overweight are risk factors for a variety of diseases, including:

- Cardiovascular disease
- Type 2 diabetes
- Deficient bone density
- Certain types of cancer

Numerous healthful foods, such as vegetables, fruits, and beans, contain fewer calories than the majority of processed foods.

A person's calorie requirements can be determined using the Dietary Guidelines.

Maintaining a healthy diet free of processed foods can assist an individual in staying within their daily calorie limit without actively monitoring their intake.

Dietary fiber is critical for weight management. Plant-based foods are high in dietary fiber, which helps regulate hunger by keeping people satisfied for longer periods.
The mayr diet, which is high in fiber and lean proteins, resulted in weight loss without requiring calorie restriction.

HOW TO GET RID OF ACID REFLUX

If you have ever suffered from heartburn, you are familiar with the sensation: a slight hiccup goes along with a burning sensation in your chest and throat.

It may be ignited by the foods you consume, particularly those that are spicy, fatty, or acidic.

Alternatively, you may suffer from gastroesophageal reflux disease (GERD), a chronic condition with numerous possible causes. Heartburn, regardless of the cause, is unpleasant and inconvenient. Acid reflux and heartburn affect millions of people.

Commercial medications, such as omeprazole, are the most frequently used treatment. However, lifestyle changes may also be beneficial.

Simply altering your dietary habits or sleeping position may significantly reduce your heartburn and acid reflux symptoms, thereby improving your quality of life.

Acid reflux occurs when stomach acid is forced up into the esophagus, the tube that connects the mouth to the stomach.
Certain types of reflux are completely normal and harmless, typically causing no symptoms. However, if this occurs frequently enough, it burns the inside of the esophagus.
In the United States, an estimated 14–20% of all adults suffer from some form of reflux.

Acid reflux's most usual symptom is heartburn, characterized by a painful, burning sensation in the chest or throat.
Around 7% of Americans, according to researchers, experience heartburn daily.

Of those who experience heartburn regularly, between 20% and 40% are diagnosed with gastroesophageal reflux disease (GERD), the most severe form of acid reflux. GERD is the most frequently occurring digestive disorder.

Additionally, reflux is frequently accompanied by an acidic taste in the back of the mouth and difficulty swallowing. Additional symptoms include a cough, asthma, tooth erosion, and sinus inflammation. **Therefore, the following are some methods for treating acid reflux and heartburn:**

1) Loose clothing
2) Erect posture
3) Erecting your upper body
4) Mixing baking soda and water simultaneously
5) Attempting ginger
6) Supplementing with licorice
7) Ingestion of apple cider vinegar
8) Chewing gum to aid in the acid dilution
9) Avoiding cigarette smoke
10) Experimenting with over-the-counter medications

Loosen clothing

Heartburn occurs when stomach contents ascend into the esophagus, where stomach acids can burn the tissue.

In some cases, you may experience heartburn as a result of tight clothing compressing your stomach.
If that is the case, the first thing you should do is unbuckle your belt — or your pants, dress, or whatever else is squeezing you.

Erect posture

Additionally, your posture can contribute to heartburn. Suppose you're seated or lying down; attempt standing. If you're already standing, try to maintain a more upright posture.
Maintaining an upright posture alleviates pressure on the lower esophageal sphincter (LES). The LES is a muscular ring that helps prevent stomach acid from rising into the esophagus.

Erecting your upper body

Lying down can aggravate heartburn. When it's time to sleep, raise your upper body by adjusting your sleeping surface.
According to the Mayo Clinic, simply raising your head with additional pillows is frequently

insufficient. Rather than that, the objective should be to elevate your body from the waist up.
If you have an adjustable bed, adjust it to a comfortable angle. If your bed is not adjustable, you can use a wedge pillow to alter the angle of your sleeping surface.

Mixing baking soda and water simultaneously.

Without discovering it, you may already have a heartburn remedy on hand in your kitchen. By neutralizing your stomach acid, baking soda can help alleviate some episodes of heartburn.
This can be accomplished by dissolving a teaspoon of baking soda in a glass of water and slowly drinking it. Indeed, you should consume all liquids slowly if you have heartburn.

Attempting ginger

For many years ago, ginger has been used as a folk remedy for heartburn. Because ginger can help with nausea, some believe it may be worth a try for heartburn as well.

Consider incorporating grated or diced ginger root into your favorite stir-fry, soup, or other recipes. To make ginger tea, dried ginger root, or ginger tea bags, steep raw ginger root in warming water.

However, it is probably best to avoid ginger ale. Carbonated beverages are a common cause of heartburn, and most ginger ale brands contain artificial flavoring.

Supplementing with licorice

Licorice root is another traditional remedy for heartburn. It is believed that it may help increase the mucous coating of the esophageal lining, thereby protecting it from stomach acid damage.

DGL is a supplement that contains licorice that has been processed to remove the majority of the glycyrrhizin, a compound that can cause adverse side effects.

Consuming an excessive amount of licorice or DGL may result in an increase in blood pressure, a decrease in potassium levels, and an interaction with certain medications. Consult your physician before taking licorice or DGL supplements.

Ingestion of apple cider vinegar

Some people use apple cider vinegar as a home remedy for heartburn to act as a buffer for stomach acid.

According to one researcher, drinking diluted apple cider vinegar after a meal may help some people with heartburn. These effects have not been statistically significant, indicating that further research is required.

If you choose to try this remedy, dilute the apple cider vinegar with water and drink it immediately after eating.

Chewing gum to aid in the acid dilution

Chewing gum for 30 minutes after meals may also help with heartburn relief.
Chewing gum stimulates the creation of saliva and the ability to swallow. It may assist in diluting and clearing stomach acid from the esophagus.

Avoiding cigarette smoke

You're probably aware that smoking is harmful to your health. However, did you know that smoking can aggravate heartburn? If you are a smoker and experience heartburn, refrain from lighting.
While smoking may be a go-to coping strategy when you're feeling uneasy, it will not alleviate the burning sensation.

Experimenting with over-the-counter medications

There are numerous over-the-counter (OTC) medications available to treat heartburn. These medications are classified into three categories:

- antacids
- H2 receptor antagonists

- proton pump inhibitors (PPIs)

PPIs and H2 blockers lessen the amount of acid secreted by the stomach, which can help prevent and alleviate heartburn symptoms. Antacids act as a buffer for stomach acid.

The summary

When heartburn strikes, numerous over-the-counter medications, home remedies, and lifestyle modifications may provide relief.

Adjusting your daily habits may also help prevent the onset of heartburn symptoms. **For instance, attempt to:**

- ✓ Stay away from common causes of heartburn, such as fatty and spicy foods
- ✓ Consume food at least three hours before bedtime
- ✓ Avoid lying down immediately after eating
- ✓ Keep a healthy weight

Consult your doctor if you experience heartburn more than twice or three times per week. They may prescribe medications or other treatments in some instances.

RECOMMENDED AND NOT RECOMMENDED FOODS IN THE DIET

A typical day at Viva Mayr might begin with quinoa porridge or spelled bread for breakfast, vegetable soup, fish, green vegetables for lunch, and a light and easily digestible dinner of fish, soup, and/or cooked vegetables for dinner. The method is free of gluten and dairy. Likewise, heavily processed and low-fat foods are unhealthy.

The Mayr Method places a premium on alkaline foods, which produce a higher pH when digested. Foods such as fruits, vegetables, nuts, and seeds fall into this category. Additionally, heart-healthy fats, gluten-free grains, and lean meat, fish, and poultry are encouraged.

Dietary guidelines change in response to scientific advances, making it difficult to stay current on current recommendations and know what to eat.

We examine current dietary recommendations and explain how to construct a diet using the mayr plan.

The mayr diet satisfies all of an individual's nutritional requirements. Humans require a certain number of calories and nutrients to maintain their health.

A balanced diet provides an individual with all the nutrients he or she requires without exceeding the daily recommended calorie intake.
By eating a balanced diet, individuals can obtain the nutrients and calories they require while abstaining from junk food and foods devoid of nutritional value.
Previously, recommended a food pyramid to the US Department of Agriculture (USDA). However, as nutritional science advances, they now recommend consuming foods from each of the five food groups and assembling a balanced plate.

The USDA recommends that half of a person's plate be composed of fruits and vegetables.
The remaining half should be grains and protein. They recommend that each meal be accompanied

by a serving of low-fat dairy or another source of daily nutrients.

The five food groups

Foods from these five groups are included in a healthy, balanced diet:

- Vegetables
- Fruits
- Grains
- Protein
- Dairy

Vegetables

Vegetables are divided into five categories:

- Leafy greens
- Red or orange vegetables
- Starchy vegetables
- Beans and peas (legumes)
- Other vegetables, such as eggplant or zucchini

People should eat a variety of veggies to receive essential nutrients and avoid dietary monotony.

In addition, the USDA suggests that adults consume vegetables from each of the five categories at least once a week.

Vegetables can be eaten raw or prepared. It's crucial to note, though, that heating vegetables reduce their nutritional content. Furthermore, some cooking methods, such as deep-frying, might result in unhealthy fats in a dish.

Fruits

The mayr diet, like any other well-balanced diet, includes plenty of fruit. However, nutritionists recommend eating entire fruits rather than drinking fruit juice.

Juice is deficient in nutrients. Furthermore, due to additional sugar, the production process frequently adds useless calories. Instead of syrup, people should eat fresh or frozen fruits or fruits canned in water.

Grains

There are two types of grains which are whole grains and refined grains.

The bran, germ, and endosperm are all elements of the grain that make up whole grains. Because the body slowly metabolizes whole grains, they have a minimal effect on blood sugar levels.

Furthermore, whole grains are higher in fiber and protein than refined grains.

The three original components are not present in refined grains since they have been treated. As a result, refined grains are significantly lower in protein and fiber, as well as causing blood sugar increases.

Grains used to be at the bottom of the government-approved dietary pyramid, which meant grains accounted for most of a person's daily caloric intake. However, according to the latest recommendations, grains should account for only a quarter of a person's plate.

At least half of a person's daily calorie intake should come from whole grains. Whole grains that are good for you include:

- Quinoa
- Oats
- Brown rice

- Barley
- Buckwheat

Protein

According to the Dietary Guidelines, everyone should eat nutrient-dense protein regularly. Based on the current standards, this protein should account for a quarter of a person's plate.

Proteins that are good for you include:

- Lean beef and pork
- Chicken and turkey
- Fish
- Beans, peas, and legumes

Dairy

Calcium can be found in dairy and enriched soy products. When possible, the USDA recommends eating low-fat alternatives.

Dairy and soy products with low-fat content include:

- Ricotta or cottage cheese
- Low-fat milk
- Yogurt

- Soy milk

Lactose intolerant people can choose low-lactose or lactose-free products or soy-based calcium and other nutritional sources.

USEFUL TIPS FOR SHOPPING

Many of us may benefit from a few basic reminders on how to purchase wisely. As many of you are aware, I developed an obsession with shopping (by shopping until I drop') to the point where it became a dilemma for me (my shopping started to become compulsive). I knew I needed to build a healthier relationship with shopping, and I did it for over a year. I don't buy as much these days, but I know what makes a great shopping trip. Allow me to share my top 10 shopping recommendations with you. I hope these are useful in your shopping endeavors.

Do not simply hop in your car and drive to your preferred shopping destination!

Take a few moments to get acquainted with this list of smart shopping tactics.

❖ **Shop with a list**.

It is my number one recommendation for a reason. Because if not planned correctly, many people overpay or buy goods they don't desire, don't need, or will never use. It is your hard-earned money and valuable time; don't you think it's worth a few minutes of preparation? Yes, it is (and remember, you are deserving of it!). So, before you go shopping, make sure you're ready. Examine what you already own - in your closet, cupboards, house, or garage – and make a note of the 'gaps' you have and the needs this item will meet. Please make sure they're true necessities rather than frivolous desires (there's a big difference). Finally, remember to take that list with you when you go shopping! Scrumpled up at the bottom of your luggage or shoved into your pocket, that list will be useless. Please make use of it and only purchase items from the list!

❖ **Set a budget**

It is critical. Many people overspend on goods they don't want, need, or use because they don't have any spending limits — they go 'all out. It is not a wise approach to shop. Set an approximate figure (or a more accurate figure if you have detailed research on what you're shopping for to back it up) for how much you'll spend on this trip, what you're comfortable spending, and what makes sense spending on this shopping trip. You want to remember this shopping trip long after the ink on the receipt has faded, right? One approach to do this is to make sure you don't spend more money than you have. As with the list, establish a budget and adhere to it! Stop purchasing once you've reached your budget, whether it's $50, $500, or $50000.

❖ **Pay with cash.**

The research is detailed: when we shop with magic plastic, whether it's a credit or debit card, we pay 20 to 50 percent more. Something about that magical plastic makes us feel like we're dealing with Monopoly money or play money. It's as though it's not real. Those credit card fees, unfortunately, are very real! So, once you've made your list and established a reasonable budget that you can keep to, take out cash and use it only for this shopping excursion. Paying with cash feels more "real," and that's exactly what we're after: to reacquaint you with the shopping experience so you only buy what you truly need and will use. As a result, you'll save a lot of money, and those impulse purchases will be much less appealing!

❖ **Set a timeframe**

Allowing yourself to wander around a shopping center is not a good idea. Many people spend their time shopping in a leisurely manner while away an afternoon in their favorite mall. It is not a method I would recommend or support. It isn't the place to go if you want to shop intelligently — no meandering! Set a time limit for yourself to finish your shopping, and when that time is up, it's time to go home. Stop shopping once you've bought all you need (and nothing you don't), and focus on something else for the rest of the day.

❖ **Pick the best time for you.**

If you don't shop at a time that works for you, it can be a tiring and unpleasant experience. Shopping when malls and businesses are busiest (such as late at night or on Saturday mornings) can result in purchasing fatigue, leaving you argumentative and irritated - hardly a state conducive to smart shopping. Remember that our physical environment impacts us, and dense, packed places, such as crowded retail malls, rarely bring out the best people. So choose a time to buy when you are at your most attentive and optimistic. To avoid being exhausted, take frequent pauses or shop for shorter periods.

❖ **Shop alone.**

Many people believe that their shopping companions are more equivalent to criminal collaborators! They can persuade us to buy things we don't desire or need, and they may have their own (often hidden) objectives for urging us to shop. Maybe they're competitive, or maybe they want to live vicariously via us and our purchases. Whatever else is going on in the other person's life, they don't have to deal with the consequences of your purchase; only you do. It's fine if you want to go shopping as a social activity, but keep it strictly social with no purchasing allowed. Visit the store or grab a bite to eat with friends, but refrain from purchasing anything until you're ready to go shopping alone.

❖ **Don't shopping when you are exhausted, hungry, emotional, frustrated, or angry.**

It isn't a full list of the emotions that drive some individuals to overshop and buy stuff they don't desire or need. They are, nevertheless, some of the most typical emotional triggers that cause people to buy unknowingly and, as a result, ineffectively. If you are exhausted, hungry, lonely, bored, or upset, you should not go shopping. Do something else until you're in a better emotional place.

❖ **Ask, "where will I wear this?"**

Too many of us make rash purchases without considering what we'll do with them. As a result, our hard-earned money and even more valuable time are being squandered on items that have no place in our closets, houses, or lives. Imagine you already own the thing you're considering purchasing to break the impulse buying loop. Fast forward through the 'thrill of the kill' and assume that this thing, the one you are holding right now, is yours: you bought it, and it is now yours. Imagine it in your closet or at home, and see it with your own eyes. Consider this: are you still enthusiastic about it? Or has it lost a little (or a lot) of its luster? So many of us don't take the time to examine if we need anything, and as a result, we wind up bringing stuff home that we never use; what a waste of time!

- **Remember that the salesperson is there to sell to you!**

No matter how kind or pleasant a salesperson is, one thing is certain: they're there to make a deal. Yes, they may be concerned that you only leave with products that you like and will use. They do, however, expect you to leave with something. That is why they are there: to sell you something or to maintain a relationship with you so that you return. That is their prerogative. Salespeople aren't there to be our friends, no matter how nice and helpful they are. They may reasonably interact with us, but their goal is to sell us something. Keep this in mind so you only buy things you need and will use, not because a persuasive salesperson persuaded (or guilted) you to do so.

- **Don't buy it just because it's on sale.**

The term "sale" is indeed a four-letter word! It is possible when accompanied with the phrase 'shoe,' is responsible for more impulsive shopping than nearly any other word! Remember that a bargain isn't a bargain if it's not for you, doesn't fit well, you don't enjoy it, or it doesn't fill a true need you have. Spending $20 on a blouse, shoes, make-up, a DVD, scented candles, a Batman clock, or anything else you'll never wear (or only wear once) is a waste of money. We rationalize it by saying, "Oh, it's on sale, it's only $20," yet $20 adds up quickly. You wouldn't throw $20 out the window, so don't throw your money away on products that look to be a "deal" owing to their reduced sale price. Only purchase things on sale if they are on your shopping list and are within your budget.

HOW CAN EXERCISE INCREASE WEIGHT LOSS?

Increased physical activity increases the number of calories your body burns for energy or "burns off" while you're dieting. A "calorie deficit" occurs when you burn calories through physical activity while also consuming fewer calories. It results in weight loss. Physical activity is beneficial to your health in general, but even more so if you're attempting to lose or maintain a healthy weight.

Traditional food ideas are combined with everyday routines in this diet plan. Mayr Method has shown to be highly simple and beneficial for Rebel and many other dieters. In the long run, adopting a mindful eating approach can help you maintain your weight loss. In addition, there are fewer risks of missing out on a nutrient or consuming fad foods because the diet incorporates a little bit of each major food group.

After all, is said and done, remember that the diet works best when you follow the rule of moderation. Most of the Mayr diet's ideas and regulations are harmless as long as you understand the basics: be more aware of what you eat, how you digest it, and how you taste it.

Exercise directly impacts our eating patterns, so we have an easier time selecting healthier choices over time when we exercise. However, dieters find it difficult to maintain rapid dietary habits, especially if they result in calorie limits if they do not exercise. Furthermore, the longer we make healthy choices, the more likely they will become second nature.

However, this approach ignores the fact that people can vary their exercise ability. For example, the ability to shed weight with exercise varies substantially as an otherwise sedentary individual's exercise capacity approaches a lean person.

It's the equivalent of handing a bucket or even a hose to the participant in our pool-emptying scenario. The ability to jog for 30 minutes or ride a bike for 60 minutes distinguishes many would-be dieters from their lean counterparts. It accounts for the majority of tried and failed weight-loss initiatives. Furthermore, if a person reaches a critical level of exercise capacity, the experience of exercising becomes more pleasurable, and it can even be enjoyable.

Is it possible to lose weight by exercising? Absolutely. Of course, rapid calorie limits will cause weight loss in the short term, but it is exceedingly difficult for people to sustain that restriction for long periods, and most people will either quit or gain back the weight they lost. Exercise, on the other hand, is a tried-and-true method of making dietary adjustments more bearable. Furthermore, focusing on exercise and increasing exercise capacity initially makes it easier to make better food choices and live a healthy lifestyle, resulting in significant weight loss that can be sustained over time.

Physical exercise program

A customized workout program tailored to your unique needs is an excellent approach to staying physically and mentally fit. It also has other advantages, including bettering the condition of the heart and lungs. In addition, muscle strength, endurance, and motor fitness have all improved. Programs specifying a variety of physical activities and the amount of time each should be completed are commonly used in gyms, where they are typically adapted to the needs of people. Fitness instructors can devise your customized exercise regimen. Your entire exercise plan should incorporate various parts, whether you construct your fitness training program or hire a personal trainer. Include cardiovascular fitness, weight training, core exercises, balance training, flexibility, and stretching in your workout routine. Five basic movements have evolved as a result of human evolution, and they comprise practically all of our daily actions." In other words, your workout requires five movements, one from each of the following categories: push (pushing away from you), pull (tugging toward you), hip-hinge (bending from the middle), squat (knee flexion), and plank.

There is no single workout that can meet all of your requirements. To get the most out of your regimen, you should do various activities throughout the week. Otherwise, it's like eating fruit—healthy in the short term solely, but devoid of many of the nutrients found in other meals like fish, veggies, nuts, and whole grains.

So, what does a well-balanced fitness routine entail?

<u>It is recommended that all individuals incorporate the following types of exercise into their weekly routines:</u>

- Three hours of moderate aerobic activity per week (for example, 30 minutes five days a week) or 75 minutes of strong aerobic activity per week.

- Two or more strength training sessions per week, with at least 48 hours between each exercise, allow muscles to recover.
- Balance exercises for older adults who are at risk of falling.

If all of this seems daunting, keep in mind that workouts can be broken down into smaller chunks. Three 10-minute walks, for example, can help you meet your daily target of 30 minutes of cardiovascular activity.

A short warm-up at the start and a cool-down at the end of each activity should be included. Gentle exercise, such as marching in place, should be used to loosen up your muscles and get more oxygen-rich blood flowing to them during the warm-up. Slow down your activity and intensity for five to ten minutes to cool down, then end with stretches to avoid stiffness.

Continue reading to learn more about each component of a well-balanced exercise regimen, as well as a variety of activities and exercises to get you started.

To get the best out of your walks, follow these tips:

- **Find a safe place to walk.**

Quiet streets with sidewalks, park trails, athletic tracks at nearby schools, and shopping malls are frequently excellent choices.

- **Buy a good pair of shoes.**

Look for soles that are supportive but flexible and cushion your feet. When it comes to walking shoes, comfort is paramount. Shopping is best done at the end of the day when your feet are at their largest. Select footwear with a "breathable" upper, such as nylon mesh.

- **Dress for comfort and safety.**

Wear less clothing than you would if you were standing motionless. Dress in layers to allow for easy removal of clothing if you become too hot. Drivers are more likely to spot you if you wear light-colored clothing and wear a luminous vest.

- **Do a five-minute warm-up and cool-down.**

For your warm-up, go at a slower pace. Slow down near the end of your stroll to cool down (even if you aren't hot). Exercise, according to experts, has no magic: you get out of it what you put in. That does not imply that you must exercise for several hours each day. All that implies is that you'll have to work smarter. Experts agree, however, that not all exercises are created equal. Some are just more effective than others, whether they target various muscle areas, are appropriate for a wide range of fitness levels, or aid in calorie burn.

- **Walking**

Cardiovascular activity, which strengthens the heart and burns calories, should be included in any fitness routine. On the other hand, walking is something you can do anywhere, at any time, with nothing more than a nice pair of shoes. It's also not just for beginners: Walking may provide a decent exercise for even the fittest individuals. According to Robert Gotlin, DO, director of orthopedic and sports rehabilitation at Beth Israel Medical Center in New York, "a fast walk can burn up to 500 calories each hour." Because it takes 3,500 calories to lose a pound, you'd lose a pound for every seven hours you walk if you didn't do anything else. However, don't go from sitting on the couch to walking for an hour in one day. Beginners should begin by walking for five to ten minutes, gradually increasing to at least 30 minutes every session.

"Don't go above five minutes at a time." Another piece of advice is to increase the length of your walks before increasing the speed or incline.

- **Interval training**

If you're a beginner or a seasoned distance runner, a walker, or an aerobic dancer, incorporating interval training into your cardiovascular routine will improve your fitness and help you lose weight.

"varying your tempo throughout the exercise session promotes the aerobic system to adapt." "The more powerful your aerobic system is, the more calories you can burn."

Pushing the intensity or tempo for a minute or two, then easing off for two to ten minutes, is the way to go (depending on how long your total workout will be and how much time you need to recover). Carry going like this for the duration of the workout.

Some other examples of physical activity are:

- Riding a bike or running (join our indoor walking program).
- Performing household chores.
- Taking the stairs rather than the elevator.
- Having fun at the park.
- Shoveling snow or raking leaves.

Importance of a Physical Exercise Programme

Summer is here, even though the weather hasn't fully arrived yet. Many individuals will be thinking about shorts, sundresses, and swimsuits as they plan adventures in the sun and vacations overseas. For some, the prospect of another thrilling summer will take them to the gym, where they will most certainly set objectives to be in shape for the season. On the other hand, fitness goals and routines can be notoriously difficult to stick to 'New Year, New Me,' especially if you don't have a lot of time before your summer adventures begin. So, how can you make sure you don't get off track? According to our fitness experts at Simply Gym Cwmbran, building a personal training program is the key to attaining your summer fitness goals.

GUIDE TO LOSING WEIGHT AND IMPROVING HEALTH

Weight Loss

There are natural ways to lose weight if your doctor suggests it. A constant weight loss of 1 to 2 pounds per week is advised for the most effective long-term weight management. However, many eating strategies will leave you hungry or unsatisfied. These are some of the primary reasons why sticking to a better eating plan may be difficult. However, not all diets have this effect. Low-carbohydrate, low-calorie diets promote weight loss and may be easier to adhere to than other types of diets. Because food equals calories, you must either eat fewer calories, exercise more to burn off calories through activity or do both to lose weight. Fat is stored as a result of food that is not utilized to power the body. One of the most important guidelines for weight loss is to make healthier food choices. Here's how:

- **Limit non-nutritious foods, such as:**
    - Sugar, honey, syrups, and candy

- Pastries, donuts, pies, cakes, and cookies
- Soft drinks, sweetened juices, and alcoholic beverages

- **Cut down on high-fat foods by:**
  - Choosing poultry, fish, or lean red meat as a protein source
  - Cooking with low-fat methods like baking, broiling, steaming, grilling, and boiling
  - Using dairy products that are low in fat or fat-free
  - Dressing salads with vinaigrette, herbs, lemon, or fat-free dressings
  - Steer clear of fatty meats, including bacon, sausage, franks, ribs, and luncheon meats.
  - Staying away from high-fat snacks such as nuts, chips, and chocolate
  - Limiting your intake of fried food
  - Reducing the amount of butter, margarine, oil, and mayonnaise used
- **Eat a variety of foods, including:**
  - Raw, steamed, or baked fruits and vegetables

- Whole grains, bread, cereals, rice, and pasta.
- Fat-free milk or yogurt, low-fat cottage cheese, and low-fat cheese.
- Protein, such as chicken, turkey, fish, lean meat, and legumes or beans

- **Change your eating habits:**
  - To help control your hunger, eat three well-balanced meals each day.
  - Eat small portions of a variety of meals and watch your portion amounts.
  - Snack on low-calorie foods
  - Only eat when you're hungry and stop when you're full.
  - Eat slowly and try not to multitask while doing so.
  - Find alternative ways to divert your attention away from food, such as going for a walk, learning a new activity, or volunteering in your community.
  - Make regular exercise a part of your daily routine.

- If you need emotional support in your weight loss efforts, join a support group.

Improving health

We've all had those good-intentioned times when we vow to make major lifestyle changes: Stop smoking. 20-pound weight loss Join a gym and begin working out every day. While we should constantly aspire to achieve these health goals, improving health doesn't always have drastic changes. Additionally, you can take several minor steps to improve your overall health and quality of life — and because they are easy to incorporate into your daily routine, they will be easy to maintain over time. Also, if you have got a few minutes to spare, this activity may be beneficial. Incorporate the activities and tactics listed below into your daily routine. When these small changes become habits, they can have a significant impact on your overall health.

- **Enjoy de-stressing.**

Stress can be reduced via regular exercise, meditation, and breathing methods, according to experts. Listening to relaxing music, reading a good book, sitting in a hot tub, or playing with your pet can all help you relax. Long-term stress can cause or exacerbate various diseases, including heart disease, stroke, high blood pressure, depression, ulcers, irritable bowel syndrome, migraines, and obesity, to name a few. Do you have a limited amount of time? Could you not get too worked up over it? Even brief bouts of relaxation, like exercise, are good. Even 10 minutes a day spent doing something you enjoy will help you cope with the stresses of regular life. Just one chapter of a book or a few laps around the block with your dog will make you feel calmer, more refreshed, and rejuvenated. If you can't take a complete break from what you're doing right now, consider taking a few slow, deep breaths. It is easier to relax when you slow down your breathing. This relaxation reaction causes the release of stress-relieving hormones in the body, increasing immunological function. Your resting heart rate can also be reduced by deep breathing. People who have lower resting heart rates are in greater physical shape than those who have higher rates.

- **Put away the salt.**

  With a saltshaker on the table, it is all too easy to digest too much salt, leading to hypertension. Therefore, store the shaker in a cabinet or pantry and use it only when cooking.

  Additionally, it is a good idea to taste your food before salting it. You may discover that it does not require any additional work. You can also season your food with lemon or lime juice, garlic, red pepper flakes, herbs, or a salt-free seasoning blend. Supply your refrigerator and pantry with your favorite fresh and dried herbs, so they're always ready to flavor your food.

- **Get to bed earlier.**

  The majority of us do not receive the seven to eight hours of sleep that adults require. A lack of sleep, regardless of your age, weight, or exercise habits, can increase your risk of a heart attack or stroke over time. If you're having trouble sleeping, even going to bed 15 minutes earlier each night can help. Establish and stick to a regular sleep and waking pattern, even on days off.

- **Have a glass of red wine.**

  The potent antioxidants present in red wine have been shown to protect against heart disease, colon cancer, anxiety, and depression in studies. Drink that glass of merlot with your evening meal – you may even use it to toast to your excellent health. But, as always, drink in moderation. While a small amount of red wine provides health benefits, excessive alcohol consumption, even red wine, may lead to a variety of health issues, including liver and kidney disease, as well as cancer. Women, in particular, must exercise caution when it comes to alcohol use. They have a higher overall risk of liver problems than men. Therefore they are more likely to develop liver problems than drink less. Two drinks per day are unlikely to hurt a healthy male; women, on the other hand, should reduce themselves to one alcoholic beverage per day.

- **Check your posture and ergonomics.**

  Take a moment to consider your posture the next time you're at your desk or on the phone. Then, with your legs uncrossed, straighten your back, tuck in your stomach, and place your feet flat on the floor. You'll immediately feel more at ease.

  One of the common health issues is back pain and a leading cause of disability.

  If you work at a computer, consider your workstation's ergonomics. How people fit and move within their environment contributes to reducing back and neck strain, carpal tunnel syndrome, eye strain, and other occupational problems. A few easy changes, including adjusting your computer monitor, switching to a chair with additional low back support, and taking regular pauses throughout the day to conduct stretching exercises, can go a long way toward making your office healthier and more pleasant.

- **Do a crossword puzzle.**

  Reading, crossword puzzles, Sodoku, and chess are among the mentally challenging activities discovered by Rush University researchers to have a protective effect on the brain.

  Regularly engaging your mind, according to research, may help lessen your risk of dementia associated with Alzheimer's disease.

  Do you dislike puzzles and games? Don't worry; there are other ways to keep your brain in good shape. Use your non-dominant hand to eat. Take a different path home from work. Connect with others as well as staying socially active may help to prevent dementia.

- **Weigh in.**

  Appropriate nutrition can help prevent heart disease, stroke, and certain types of cancer. But there's another incentive for women to avoid gaining weight: it lowers the likelihood of future pelvic floor diseases.

  Women who have had their babies vaginally are more likely to have pelvic floor issues. According to a recent study, even women who have never given birth vaginally are more likely to develop urinary stress incontinence if they are overweight or obese.

- **Make a few dietary substitutions.**
  - Opt for whole-grain alternatives to white bread, rice, crackers, and pasta.
  - Use skinless chicken and turkey instead of skin-on, as well as leaner cuts of beef or pork in your dishes.

- Replace one sugary beverage (soda, juice, etc.) with a tall glass of water each day.
- Instead of reaching for candy bars or potato chips, nibble on a handful of almonds or walnuts, a piece of the whole apple, or carrot sticks dipped in hummus between meals.

Additionally, try to include an additional serving of nonstarchy veggies in your daily diet. Do you want something to eat? Instead of a cookie, eat a carrot. Are you preparing a meal for your family? Instead of mashed potatoes, serve broccoli or spinach as a side dish. Green peas or red or yellow pepper slices can be added to brown rice or sandwich pieces. Vegetables, especially dark, leafy greens, are well-known for their health benefits. However, there is an additional advantage to including more vegetables in your regular diet: They're high in fiber and water, which means they'll keep you full and satisfied without adding too many calories or fat to your diet. There are tons of great recipes in cookbooks and online for excellent and healthy veggie dishes, including Rush's content center.

- **Take the stairs.**

  When you need to get to a higher floor, skip the elevator and use the stairs instead. You'll get your blood pumping, your lungs working, and your lower body muscles working. It's a fantastic way to fit some exercise into your day without having to schedule it.

  Taking the stairs counts toward your daily step total if you're aiming for the necessary 10,000 steps. These minor changes might add up to a healthier you.

- **Stretch it out.**

  Stretching your muscles regularly can help you avoid injuries, stay limber, and move freely as you age. Before and after your workout, spend a few minutes stretching. Take a few stretch breaks if you aren't working exercise that day. Look for a peaceful area in the office where you won't be interrupted. Are you on the go? Look for opportunities to stretch in your everyday routine, such as stepping out of the car or reaching for products on a high shelf at the shop. Stretching shortly before bed might also help you relax and fall asleep faster.

7-DAY EATING PLAN TO LOSE EXCESS WEIGHT

It isn't a crash diet: you'll consume three meals and two snacks every day, with each dish including a satisfying ratio of 45 percent carbohydrates, 30 percent protein, and 25 percent healthy fats. Forberg suggests sticking to no- and low-calorie beverages like coffee, tea, and water when it comes to liquids. And The Biggest Loser trainer Bob Harper recommends doing 60 to 90 minutes of moderate activity four times a week to speed up weight loss and develop a healthy and strong body.

Monday

Breakfast:

- 1/2 cup egg whites, one teaspoon olive oil, one teaspoon basil, one teaspoon grated Parmesan, and 1/2 cup cherry tomatoes scrambled
- One whole-grain bread piece
- 1 cup blueberries
- 1 cup of skim milk

Snack:

- 1/4 cup sliced strawberries on top of 1/2 cup fat-free Greek yogurt

Lunch:

Three-quarter (3/4) cup cooked bulgur, 4 ounces chopped grilled chicken breast, 1 tbsp shredded low-fat cheddar, diced grilled veggies (2 tsp onion, 1/4 cup diced zucchini, 1/2 cup bell pepper), 1 tsp chopped cilantro, and one tablespoon low-fat vinaigrette.

Snack:

- Six baby carrots and two tablespoons of hummus

Dinner:

- Grilled salmon
- 1 cup wild rice Plus 1 tablespoon toasted almonds, slivered
- 1 cup wilted baby spinach Plus one teaspoon olive oil plus one teaspoon balsamic vinegar Plus 1 teaspoon grated Parmesan
- 1/2 cup sliced cantaloupe
- 1 teaspoon chopped walnuts and 1/2 cup all-fruit raspberry sorbet

Tuesday

Breakfast:

- Half cup skim milk; 3/4 cup steel-cut or old-fashioned oatmeal prepared with water
- 2 country-style turkey sausage links
- 1 pound blueberries

Snack:

- 1 tsp chopped walnuts, 1/2 cup fat-free ricotta cheese, and 1/2 cup raspberries

Lunch:

- Half cup low-fat cottage cheese + 1/2 cup salsa

Dinner:

- 1 burger made of turkey
- 3/4 cup roasted broccoli and cauliflower florets
- Brown rice, 3/4 cup
- 1 tablespoon light balsamic vinaigrette on 1 cup spinach salad

Wednesday

Breakfast:

- 4 egg whites and one whole egg, one-quarter cup chopped broccoli, two tablespoons fat-free refried beans, diced onion, sliced mushrooms, and salsa in an omelet
- Quesadilla using half a small corn tortilla and one tablespoon low-fat jack cheese
- 1/2 cup watermelon, diced

Snack:

- One sliced apple and one tablespoon chopped walnuts in 1/2 cup fat-free vanilla yogurt

Lunch:

- 2 cups Romaine lettuce, 4 ounces grilled chicken, 1/2 cup chopped celery, 1/2 cup diced mushrooms, 2 tsp shredded low-fat cheddar, and 1 tsp Caesar dressing
- 1 nectarine, medium
- 1 gallon skim milk

Snack:

- 1 mozzarella string cheese stick (fat-free)
- 1 orange, medium

Dinner:

- 4 oz. Shrimp, grilled or sautéed with 1 tbsp. Olive oil and 1 tbsp. minced garlic
- 1 steamed medium artichoke
- 1 tablespoon fat-free honey mustard dressing, 1/2 cup whole wheat couscous, two teaspoons diced bell pepper, 1/4 cup garbanzo beans, 1 tsp chopped fresh cilantro

Thursday

Breakfast:

- 1 tablespoon nut butter and one tablespoon sugar-free fruit spread on a light whole-grain English muffin
- 1 honeydew wedge
- 1 gallon skim milk
- 2 slices bacon from Canada

Snack:

- 1 cup low-fat vanilla yogurt, 2 tsp sliced strawberries or raspberries, and 2 tsp low-fat granola in a yogurt parfait

Lunch:

- 4 ounces thinly sliced lean roast beef wrapped in a 6-inch whole-wheat tortilla with a quarter cup of shredded lettuce, three medium tomato slices, 1 tsp horseradish, and 1 tsp Dijon mustard
- Half-cup pinto beans or lentils with one tablespoon light Caesar dressing and one teaspoon chopped basil

Snack:

- 2 tablespoons guacamole on eight cooked corn chips (try one of these guac recipes)

Dinner:

- 4 oz. halibut, grilled
- half cup of sliced mushrooms, 1/4 cup chopped yellow onion, and 1 cup green beans cooked in 1 teaspoon olive oil
- Arugula salad with 1/2 cup halved cherry tomatoes and one teaspoon balsamic vinaigrette
- One-quarter cup fat-free vanilla yogurt + 1/2 cup warm unsweetened applesauce
- 1 tablespoon nuts, chopped, and a pinch of cinnamon

Friday

Breakfast:

- Medium whole wheat tortilla, four scrambled egg whites, 1 tsp olive oil, 1/4 cup fat-free refried black beans, two teaspoons salsa, two tablespoons grated low-fat cheddar, and one teaspoon fresh cilantro are used to make this burrito.

- 1 cup melon (mixed)

Snack:

- 3 oz. lean ham, sliced
- 1 apple, medium

Lunch:

- Burgers made of turkey (or one of these veggie burgers)
- 1 cup baby spinach, one-quarter cup halved cherry tomatoes, 1/2 cup cooked lentils, two teaspoons grated Parmesan, and one tablespoon light Russian dressing for a salad
- 1 gallon skim milk

Snack:

- 1 mozzarella string cheese stick (fat-free)
- 1 cup grapes (red)

Dinner:

- 5 oz. wild salmon, grilled
- 1/2 cup wild or brown rice
- 1 tablespoon low-fat Caesar dressing on 2 cups mixed baby greens
- 1 sliced pear and 1/2 cup all-fruit strawberry sorbet

Saturday

Breakfast:

- 3 big egg whites, two tablespoons sliced bell peppers, two teaspoons chopped spinach, two tablespoons part-skim shredded mozzarella, and two teaspoons pesto
- 1 bran muffin (small)
- 1 gallon skim milk

Snack:

- 1 tsp ground flaxseed and 1/2 cup diced pear in 1/2 cup low-fat vanilla yogurt

Lunch:

- 4 oz. turkey breast, sliced
- 5 tomato slices, 1/4 cup sliced cucumber, one teaspoon fresh chopped thyme, and one tablespoon fat-free Italian dressing in a tomato-cucumber salad
- 1 orange, medium

Snack:

- 3/4 cup skim milk, half banana, 1/2 cup low-fat yogurt, and 1/4 cup sliced strawberries in a smoothie (Psst: Here are more weight loss smoothie ideas.)

Dinner:

- 1 tsp olive oil, one teaspoon lemon juice, and 1/2 teaspoon no-sodium seasoning baked into 4 ounces red snapper
- 1 cup spaghetti squash, one teaspoon olive oil, two teaspoon Parmesan cheese, grated

- 1 cup green beans, cooked, with one tablespoon slivered almonds

Sunday

Breakfast:

- 2 slices bacon from Canada
- 1 sugar-free fruit spread on a whole-grain toaster waffle
- Berries, 3/4 cup
- 1 gallon skim milk

Snack:

- • 1 tsp slivered almonds, 1/4 cup fat-free cottage cheese, and 1/4 cup cherries

Lunch:

- Two cups of baby spinach, 4 ounces grilled chicken, 1 tsp chopped dried cranberries, three avocado slices, 1 tsp slivered walnuts, and two tablespoons of low-fat vinaigrette
- One apple
- 1 gallon skim milk

Snack:

- 1 tsp sugar-free fruit spread and 1 tsp ground flaxseed in 1/4 cup fat-free Greek yogurt
- A quarter cup of blueberries

Dinner:

- 4 oz. lean pork tenderloin with onions, garlic, broccoli, and bell pepper stir-fried
- A half cup of brown rice
- 1 teaspoon of sliced ginger, chopped cilantro, light soy sauce, and rice wine vinegar in 5 medium tomato slices

USEFUL TIPS

Additional weight-loss tips include the following:

- Meal and snack planning, as well as purchasing just items on the shopping list
- Maintaining an awareness of portion sizes and the ratios of various macronutrients.
- Incorporating protein and fiber into all meals.
- Experimenting with various herbs and spices to bring variety to meals and reduce the need for added sugar, salt, and fat.
- Preparing healthy meals in bulk for freezing.
- Avoiding prolonged periods of fasting to stave off cravings for unhealthy snacks.
- Maintaining adequate hydration to stave off cravings for sugary beverages.
- Engaging in 30 minutes of moderate-intensity physical activity on the majority, if not all, of the week's days.
- Associating with a diet and exercise partner.

MAYR DIET RECIPES FOR BEGINNERS AND INEXPERIENCED

1. Alkaline Recipes

You may lose weight, gain energy, enhance your metabolism, and feel younger with The Alkaline Cure-all from the comfort of your own home.

A dash of grapefruit juice adds a tangy and refreshing edge to this quinoa salad with avocado, tomato, parsley, and pine nuts recipe. While citrus fruits are acidic when consumed, they turn alkaline when digested. Who was aware?

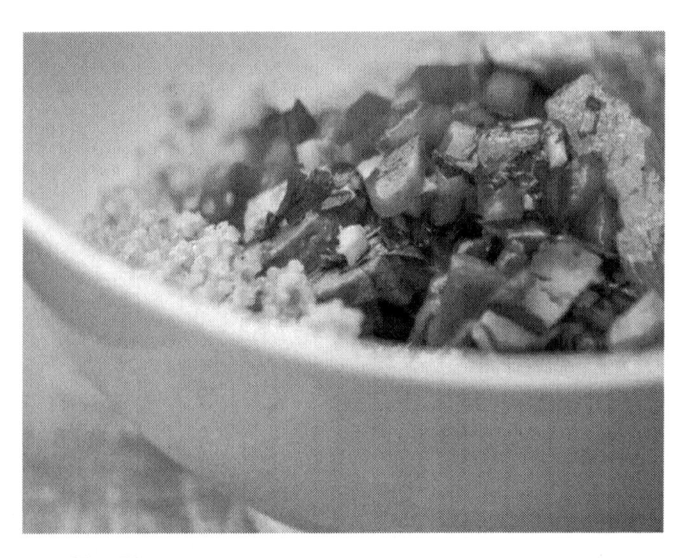

The Alkaline Cure

Is there a thing as a nutritious soup cooked with cream? Yes, it is correct! This alkaline minestrone dish can be served chunky or puréed for a creamier texture.

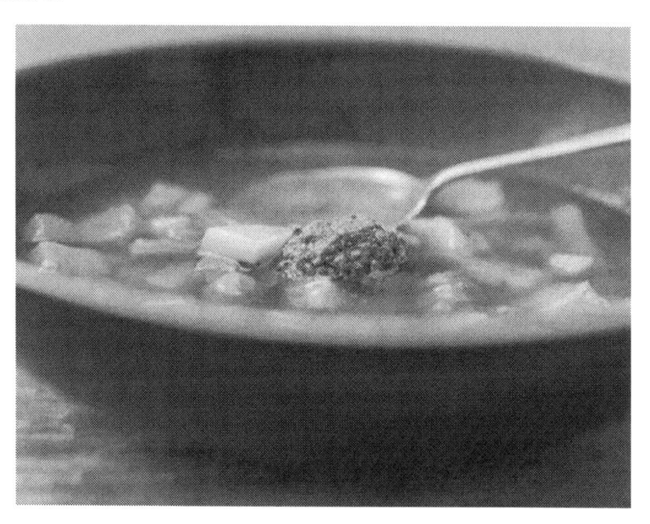

The Alkaline

For a quick and easy lunch, save the skins from baked potato with an alkaline mayonnaise recipe and fill them with curd and herbs. Spud-tacular.

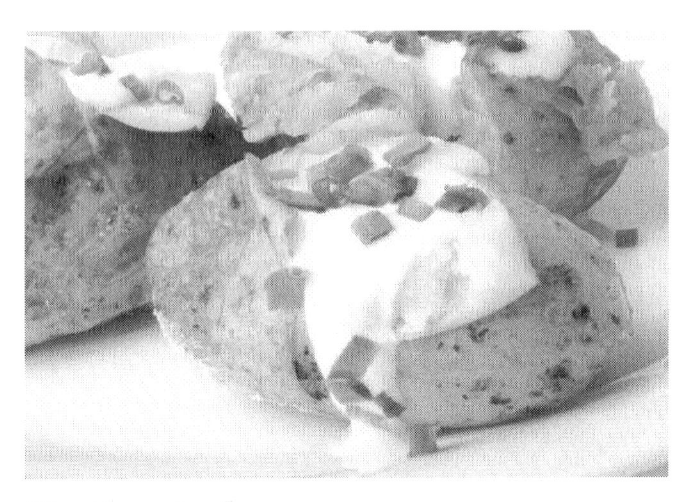

Shutter stock

2. Porridge Recipes

By now, you've probably built up a mental library of your favorite porridge recipes that you can call upon anytime the mood strikes for a satisfying and nutritious meal (no, not just breakfast).

Perhaps you have a go-to macro calculator-friendly porridge recipe for weekdays (something quick like a spoonful of nut butter and a coarsely sliced banana) and one for lazy weekends that is a little more indulgent (complete with meticulously laid toppings and the expensive fresh berries. You know the ones).

In either case, experimenting with new porridge recipes may help keep mealtimes interesting and help you integrate new nutrients into your diet by varying the toppings and flavorings. That is the question: to add protein powder or not to add protein powder.

i. Baked Apple Pudding Porridge

If you enjoy porridge recipes with a homey flavor, this warm apple-based bowl is for you.

Add diced apple, a handful of raisins, and one teaspoon cinnamon powder to a cup of plain oats. If you have time, warm the apple and raisins with a small amount of honey for five minutes.

The benefits:

- **Cinnamon**

  This super-spice helps to control blood sugar levels and alleviates exhaustion.

- **Apple**

  Besides providing 14% of your daily vitamin C requirement, apple antioxidants may help increase workout endurance.

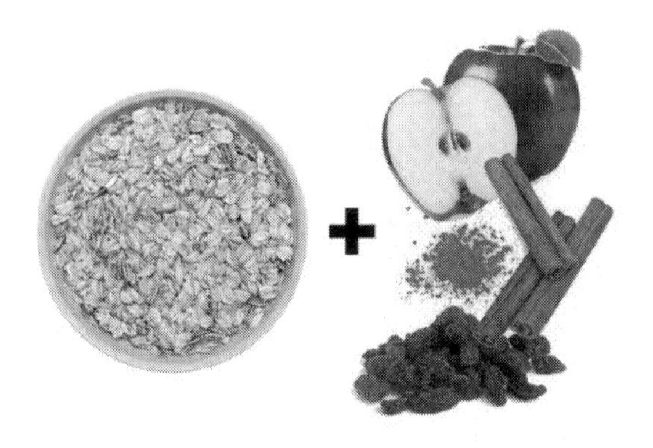

Cinnamon and Apple

ii. Banoffee Porridge Recipe

Porridge is much more than just a bowl of oats, as this banana-based dish demonstrates — and it's also an excellent pre- or post-run snack if you're training.

Simply combine a sliced banana, one teaspoon cacao nibs, and a drizzle of agave nectar in a small bowl. Yum. Porridge is much more than just a bowl of oats, as this banana-based dish demonstrates — and it's also an excellent pre- or post-run snack if you're training.

Simply combine a sliced banana, one teaspoon cacao nibs, and a drizzle of agave nectar in a small bowl. Yum.

<u>The benefits:</u>

- **Banana**

  Potassium-rich to improve muscle function and reduce cramping after exercise.

- **Cacao**

  One of the richest essential nutrients of magnesium is essential for muscle function and bone strength and which the body cannot create.

- **Agave**

  Anti-inflammatory and immune-boosting capabilities have been proven.

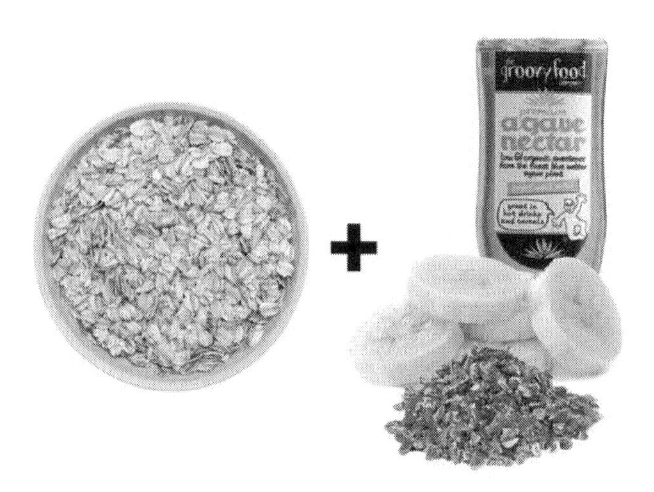

Banana, Cacao, and Agave

iii. Black Forest Gateau Porridge

If you're feeling luxurious, add a handful of fresh or dried sour cherries, one teaspoon of cacao nibs, and a dollop of Crème Fraiche.

The benefits:

- **Cherries**

  Cherries speed up muscle healing and reduce discomfort.

- **Cacao**

  For optimum muscular tone, more antioxidants than green tea or red wine are used.

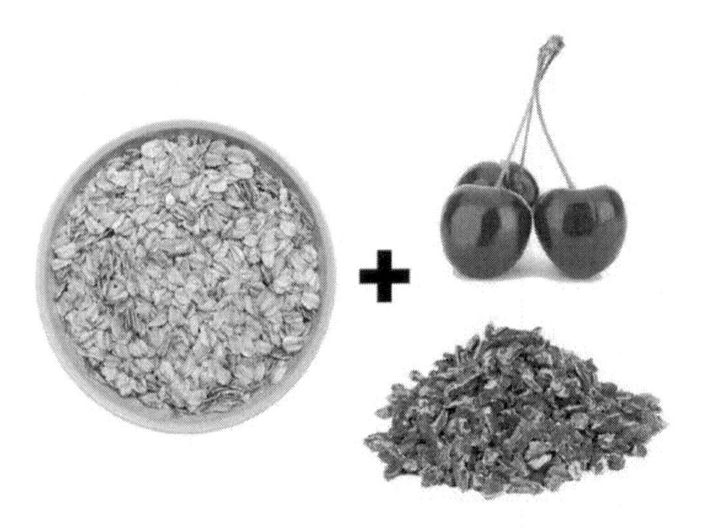

Cherries and Cacao

iv. Chai Latte Porridge

Make your oats with water and Chai Latte powder, then sprinkle 1 tsp honey and 1 tsp cinnamon powder over the top. It smells as nice as it tastes.

The benefits:

- **Chai**

  Chai contains a high concentration of antioxidants because of the black tea used.

- **Honey**

  Honey's antibacterial properties will help you get rid of sniffles and sneezes.

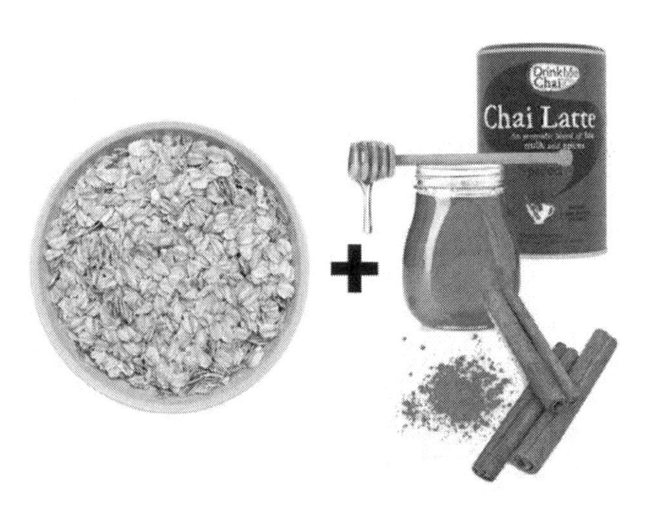

Chai and Honey

v. Pineapple Protein Porridge

Coyo coconut yogurt is used to make the porridge, which is then stirred in with pineapple pieces. Simple.

<u>The benefits:</u>

- **Coconut milk**

  Antibacterial, antifungal, and antiviral acids are found in this product.

- **Pineapple**

  This superfruit helps your body utilize protein more effectively by providing 80 percent of your daily vitamin C.

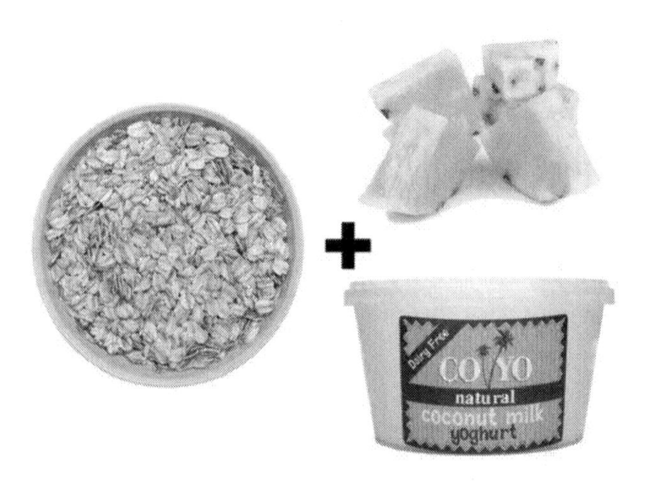

Coconut Milk and Pineapple

vi. Fig, ricotta, and honey porridge

For a creamy, sweet porridge that tastes like a summer vacation, stir in a chopped fig, 1 tbsp soft ricotta, and 1 tsp honey.

The benefits include:

- **Ricotta**

  Sweet ricotta, soft cheese with both omega-3 and omega-6 oils, is a great way to get your healthy fat fix.

- **Figs**

  This satisfying fruit lowers blood sugar levels, has the highest calcium content of any fruit and is high in fiber.

- **Honey**

  It has the exact fructose and glucose amounts needed to keep blood sugar in check.

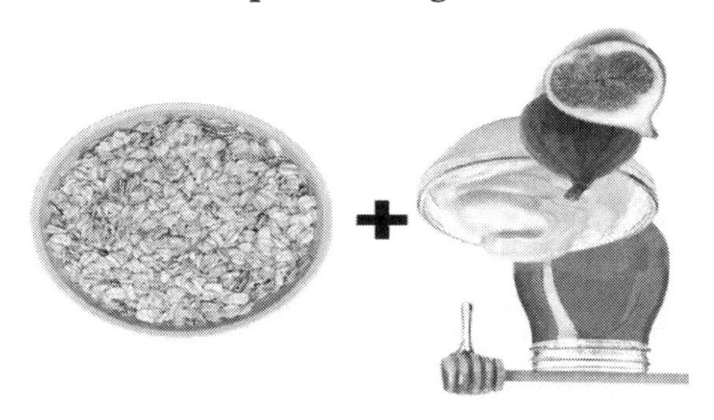

Ricotta, Figs, and Honey

vii. Healthy Nutella Porridge

Make the porridge with hazelnut milk and one tablespoon of cacao nibs. We're childish, aren't we?

The benefits include:

- **Hazelnuts**

  The combination of fiber, vitamins, and minerals results in a lower risk of cancer and disease.

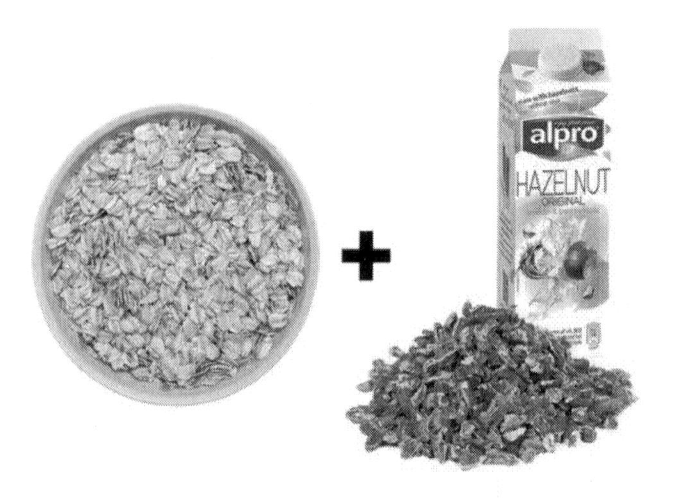

Hazelnuts

viii. Arabian Orange, Cardamom, and Date Porridge

While the porridge is boiling, toss in the whole cardamom pods, one teaspoon orange blossom honey, and a handful of sliced dates.

The benefits include:

- **Cardamom**

  It provides 175 percent of your daily iron needs, which aids in the conversion of glucose to energy, red blood cell synthesis, and workout recovery.

- **Dates**

  They're terrific energy boosters with plenty of natural sugars, plus they're cholesterol-free and low in fat.

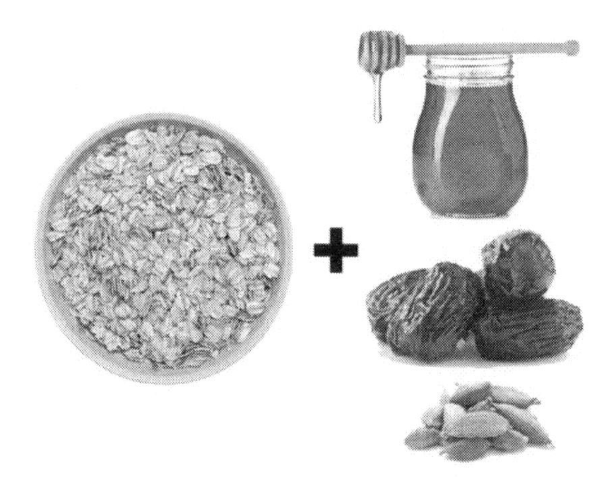

Cardamom and Dates

IX. Pecan Pie Porridge

Stir in 1 tsp maple syrup and a tiny handful of chopped pecan nuts once the porridge is done. Delicious.

The benefits include:

- **Maple syrup**

  Anti-inflammatory and antioxidant substances may aid in the prevention of diabetes, cancer, osteoporosis, and Alzheimer's disease.

- **Pecans**

  Monounsaturated fatty acids are rich in monounsaturated fatty acids, which help to decrease LDL ('bad') cholesterol.

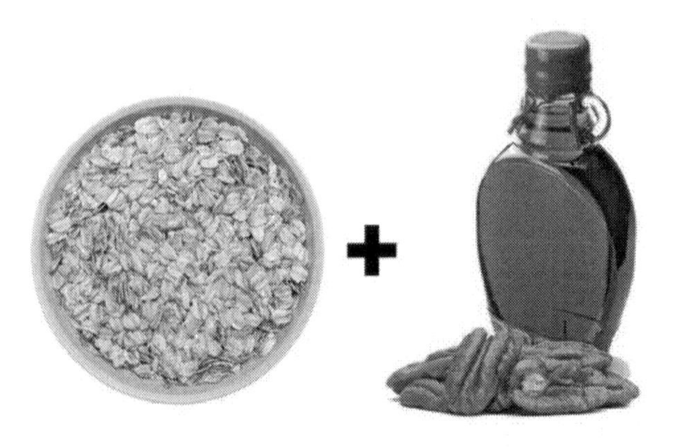

Maple Syrup and Pecans

X. Rhubarb, Pistachio, and Rose Porridge

The greek yogurt works nicely with the rhubarb in one of the most unusual porridge recipes.

1 tbsp Greek yogurt and a squirt of rosewater are all that's required. Rhubarb (stewed or compote), a handful of shelled pistachio nuts, and one teaspoon of honey are served on top. Perfect.

The benefits include:

- **Pistachios**

  Assist in the prevention of dry skin.

- **Rhubarb**

  A fourth of your daily vitamin K helps keep your complexion smooth, plus a lot of flavor for very few calories.

3. Banana Quinoa Breakfast Cups

This recipe is a one-bowl miracle that is incredibly simple to prepare. It is the perfect protein and fiber-packed recipe to use up cooked quinoa and bananas that are "on the verge" in my fridge. Make these make-ahead breakfasts/snacks your own by adding your favorite toppings and serving them cold, warm, or anywhere in between.

Note: I prefer cassava flour as a "partner flour," but if you don't have any on hand, try increasing the almond flour or substituting tapioca starch or even oatmeal flour. Play around and have fun!

Ingredients

- Two mashed bananas
- 1 tsp vanilla extract
- 1 tsp coconut sugar or honey
- Quarter cup non-dairy milk
- Half cup of almond flour
- Quarter cup cassava flour
- ½ tsp salt
- ½ tsp baking powder
- One cup cooked (and cooled) quinoa
- Two tsp chia seeds

Blueberries, chocolate chips, chopped almonds, nut butter, and coconut shreds are all optional toppings.

Directions

1. Mix mash the bananas and add the vanilla, coconut sugar or honey (if using), and milk. Combine the quinoa, flours, salt, baking powder, and chia seeds in a large mixing bowl.
2. Preheat the oven to 350 degrees Fahrenheit and ready the muffin pan. Allow 10-12 minutes for the chia seeds to gel before serving.
3. Fill muffin cups halfway with batter and top with desired contents.
4. Bake for 20 minutes at 350°F.
5. Cool the cups in the muffin pan before storing them in the refrigerator (or freezing them!)

Peanut Butter Chocolate Balls

Ingredients

- 1 Chocolate Protein Powder
- half cup of almond flour
- 1/4 cup natural peanut butter
- 4 tsp honey
- 2 tsp dairy-free mini chocolate chips
- water (as needed)

Directions

1. Combine the chocolate protein powder, almond flour, peanut butter, honey, and chocolate chips in a mixing bowl.
2. Slowly drizzle in the water as needed, mixing until the dough reaches the desired consistency.
3. Form dough into balls, lay on a tray, and freeze for one hour.
4. Just before removing the balls from the freezer, microwave the peanut butter that had been set aside.
5. Roll balls in peanut butter, generously coating them with gloves. Return to the freezer for 1 hour.

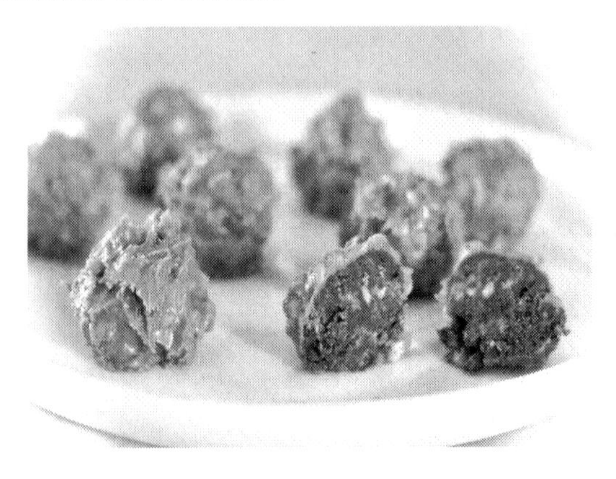

Banana Quinoa

WHEN TO EAT RAW FOOD?

Raw foods can be consumed at any time of the year. But the perfect time to eat raw is when the weather is hot and humid, and the elements have naturally increased the heat.

What kind of energy do "raw" meals have?
I'm not talking about raw dehydrated foods, raw flax crackers, or raw kale chips that have been dried and covered with various "cheese-like" stuff. I'm talking about cool-to-the-touch raw fruits and vegetables that are pouring with moisture. Consider slicing into a luscious summer peach or a cold cucumber. That's the type of raw food I'm referring to. Raw fruits and vegetables provide cooling and purifying vitality. During the scorching summer months, it's what the earth naturally gives for its inhabitants.
Summer fruits and vegetables are high in moisture, which helps to keep us cool when we eat them.
The following are some delicious examples:

- ✓ Cucumbers

- ✓ Tomatoes
- ✓ Peppers
- ✓ Bibb lettuce
- ✓ Red and green leaf lettuce
- ✓ Romaine
- ✓ Strawberries
- ✓ Blueberries
- ✓ Watermelon
- ✓ Peaches
- ✓ Plums
- ✓ Grapes

NOW is the greatest time to start that raw foods diet you've been asking me about if you're still carrying excess weight from the winter. In the winter, eating too many fresh fruits and vegetables will cool your body, slow your metabolism, and cause you to gain weight. During the hot summer months, however, the opposite occurs. Raw fruits and vegetables, with their cooling and cleaning properties, aid in weight loss. Inflammatory disorders such as heart disease, MS, Hashimoto's, and rheumatoid arthritis can all benefit from raw foods.

The body and its organs are affected energetically by the food you eat and its prepared manner.

WHEN TO EAT COOKED FOOD?

We recommend scheduling dinner approximately four to five hours after lunch. Bear in mind that if your supper time falls between 5 and 6 p.m., you will be entering the final hour of your body's high metabolic rate. Your objective is to minimize the time a food is in the "danger zone" - between 40 and 140 degrees Fahrenheit (4 and 60 degrees Celsius) — where bacteria can rapidly develop. When ready to eat, reheat leftovers on the stovetop, in a regular oven, or the microwave until the internal temperature reaches 165 degrees Fahrenheit (74 C). When you're trying to lose weight, you've undoubtedly spent a lot of time thinking about what you eat, attempting to find a balance of vegetables, carbs, fruits, and protein. However, did you know that the time you eat is as critical as the food you eat? By eating at the proper times throughout the day, you can receive a range of benefits, including weight maintenance, increased energy, and may even help you fight disease. We've included some dietary suggestions on when to consume your meals to assist you in your weight loss attempts. We've included some advice on food planning and strategies to match mealtimes with our workout regimens.

When Should You Eat Breakfast?

Breakfast, as many of us already know, is the most important meal of the day. When you eat breakfast, you establish the pattern for the remainder of the day's blood sugar levels. Consume food within the first hour following your awakening, between 6 and 10 a.m. It is the optimal interval for preparing yourself for your next meal, which should occur a few hours after breakfast.

Breakfast has a huge impact on the remainder of your day, which is why it is critical to avoid blood sugar spikes caused by pastries or sugary coffee drinks. These blood sugar swings can leave you feeling elated and depressed throughout the day. Instead, consume protein, complete grains, and healthy fats. Whole grain toast with peanut butter, eggs, and fresh fruit are just a few of the numerous nutritious options.

Eat Lunch When Your Metabolism Peaks

Each day, between 10 a.m. and 2 p.m., your metabolism reaches it's optimum, giving you enhanced digestive function and making this the optimal time to have lunch. This meal should be lighter in carbohydrate content than breakfast and dinner.

Due to the likelihood that you will be at school or work during this period, prepare your lunch the night before or order a healthy meal from a favorite local restaurant to avoid fast food and other unhealthy options.

When Should Dinner be Served?

We recommend scheduling dinner approximately four to five hours after lunch. Bear in mind that if your supper time falls between 5 and 6 p.m., you will be entering the final hour of your body's high metabolic rate. It is critical to have a longer space between your final meal of the day and your bedtime. It can assist your body in focusing on rest and renewal rather than digestion.

WHAT IS THE ROLE OF PROTEIN IN WEIGHT MANAGEMENT?

Protein is the most critical nutrient for weight loss and a more attractive body. A high protein diet increases metabolism, suppresses hunger, and alters the activity of many weight-regulating hormones. Protein's ability to repair, develop, and create muscle mass is one of its most critical functions. By reducing fat and increasing muscle mass, you can get faster metabolism, which allows for a higher calorie burn even when the body is at rest.

Protein is the single most critical nutrient for healthy weight gain. Muscle is composed of protein, and without it, the majority of those additional calories will likely be stored as body fat. According to studies, a high-protein diet causes a large portion of the excess calories to be converted to muscle when people overeat.

A sedentary adult should ingest 0.8 grams of protein per kilogram of body weight, or 0.36 grams each pound. It suggests that the average inactive man should consume approximately 56 grams of protein daily, while the average sedentary woman should consume approximately 46 grams.

Because protein contains calories, ingesting an excessive amount might make losing weight more difficult – especially if you consume protein drinks in addition to your regular diet and do not exercise. A typical adult requires between 46 and 56 grams of protein per day, depending on their weight and overall health.

For instance, higher whey protein consumption, both with and without exercise, is associated with improved weight loss, body composition, and perceived hunger in overweight and obese adults. Consuming an adequate amount of protein is critical for your health. As a result, the Daily Value (DV) for protein is set at 50 grams. According to several academics, many people should consume substantially more than this amount.

The American College of Sports Medicine (ACSM) suggests that an individual consumes between 1.2 and 1.7 g of protein per kilogram of body weight per day to grow muscle mass in conjunction with regular exercise. That's 71-100 g for a 130-lb lady aiming to increase muscle growth and strength, and 82-116 g for a 150-lb guy. According to the Institute of Medicine, all people should consume 0.83 grams of protein per kilogram of body weight each day. It equates to 56 grams for an average male and 46 grams for an average female every day.

HOW CAN WE CALM THE DIGESTIVE SYSTEM THAT GOES HAYWIRE?

Ever pondered why you get "butterflies" in your stomach when you're about to perform a strenuous task? Or why, following a fight, you feel as if your stomach is "twisted in knots"? Have you ever had an extended encounter with a toilet that wasn't induced by anything you ate? Stomach issues are a typical indication of stress and adversity.

Stress may take a physical toll on your digestive system, whether it's a single nerve-wracking event or continuous worry and stress over time. When you are stressed, some hormones and chemicals released by your body make their way into your digestive tract, where they obstruct digestion. The ensuing chemical imbalance can manifest itself in a variety of gastrointestinal disorders.

<u>The following are common gastrointestinal symptoms and conditions associated with stress:</u>

- ✓ Indigestion
- ✓ Stomach cramps
- ✓ Diarrhea

- ✓ Constipation
- ✓ Loss of appetite
- ✓ Abnormal hunger
- ✓ Nausea

Once you have one of these disorders, it can become a cause of anxiety and significantly influence your quality of life. I've seen many patients who have diarrhea develop a dread of having accidents in their trousers, making them fearful of leaving their home or going to particular areas. If you suffer from stomach cramps or indigestion, you may develop a dread of these symptoms, limiting where and what you eat, which may affect your social life.

Six Tips for Reducing Stress and Getting Things Back on Track

1. While chaos and worry are an unavoidable part of life, there is some good news. You can control your stress in such a way that it has a little effect on your stomach. Here are six strategies to help you manage stress AND the gastrointestinal difficulties that accompany it.

2. Take brief breaks and inhale deeply. When done correctly, this can be beneficial. Every couple of hours, pause for one minute and practice slow, quiet deep breathing. You're going to be astounded by the results. Breathe extremely slowly, silently, and via your nose. When you inhale, push your stomach out and allow it to deflate as you exhale.

3. Say "no." Attempting to do everything and satisfy everyone all of the time is a definite way to go awry. Recognize your boundaries and refrain from accepting new obligations when you are on the verge of exceeding them.

4. Exercise or practice yoga. Even if only for fifteen minutes a day, physical activity is an excellent way to relieve stress. When you exercise, your body releases endorphins, which connect with receptors in your brain, resulting in a pleasurable experience.

5. Rather than worrying about things you can't control, concentrate on the things you can, such as how you choose to respond to challenges. Your reaction, including how you react to gastrointestinal difficulties, is entirely up to you. Accepting stomach issues will alleviate your worry and help you manage your symptoms. Worrying about your stomach serves to exacerbate your problems.

6. Each day, listen to a guided relaxation practice. Not only will you feel relaxed while you're doing it, but the majority of people report feeling tranquil for hours afterward.

Seek the assistance of an anxiety-specialist therapist. Chronic concern and intricate anxiety are frequently too difficult to manage on your own. A good Cognitive Behavioral Therapist will know the appropriate course of action. ADAA.org can assist you in locating a therapist.

Stress and its effect on the stomach require effort to alleviate. These proposals have the potential to work if implemented appropriately and made a daily priority. Expecting immediate benefits and a complete absence of symptoms, on the other hand, will add to your frustration and problems. It is critical to accept some degree of stomach discomfort.

Finally, examine your diet. Certain foods are known to cause stomach irritation. Consult a physician and follow any medical recommendations. Numerous gastrointestinal ailments cannot be addressed only through stress reduction. When attempting to tackle gut-related issues, it is necessary to consider biological, psychological, and social factors. Each of us responds differently to stress. Regardless of how stress affects you, internalizing it can result in chronic health concerns such as heart disease, hypertension, obesity, and depression.

HOW MUCH WATER DO WE NEED?

Every day, you should aim to consume between half an ounce and an ounce of water for every pound you weigh." If you weigh 150 pounds, this equates to 75 to 150 ounces of water per day. If a survivor were to find oneself in a position where water was limited, they would undoubtedly become dehydrated, and their rate of urination would decrease to 500ml for argument's sake. It leaves an approximate number of 1 Litre or 32 ounces to sustain the average human when resting in a temperate area.

A regularly active person needs approximately three-quarters of a gallon of fluid per day from water and other liquids. Minimum Absolute Requirements. For replacement reasons, it has been calculated that a "typical" individual requires roughly 3 liters (3.2 quarts) of water per day, assuming average temperate temperature conditions.

Several reasons may require you to adjust your total fluid intake:

- **Exercise:** If you engage in any activity that causes you to sweat, you should drink additional water to compensate for the fluid loss. It is critical to consume water before, during, and after an exercise.
- **Environment:** Extremely hot or humid weather might cause excessive sweating and require more fluids intake. At high altitudes, dehydration is also a possibility.
- **Overall health:** When you have a fever, vomiting, or diarrhea, your body loses fluids. Consume additional water or, if directed by a physician, oral rehydration solutions. Additionally, bladder infections and urinary tract stones may necessitate greater fluid consumption.
- **Pregnancy and breastfeeding:** If you are pregnant or nursing, you may require additional fluids to maintain proper hydration.

WHEN DO WE NEED IT?

Water is important to digest food and eliminate waste. Water is required for the production of digestive juices, urine (pee), and feces. And you can bet that the primary component of perspiration, usually known as sweat, is water. Apart from being a critical component of the body's fluids, water is required for each cell to function properly. Thirty minutes before a meal, drink one glass of water to aid digestion. Avoid drinking too soon before or after a meal to avoid diluting the digestive fluids. Drink water an hour after eating to allow the nutrients to be absorbed by the body. Water is used by the body in every cell, organ, and tissue to assist in regulating temperature and perform other bodily activities. Because your body drains water through breathing, sweating, and digesting, it is vital to rehydrate with drinks and water-containing foods. As a general rule, a human can survive for around three days without water. However, some factors, such as the amount of water required by an individual body and how it uses it, might change this. Water nourishes all of our cells, particularly muscle cells, delaying muscular weariness. 2. Water contributes to weight loss. Water helps you feel fuller for longer without adding calories. If you're unsure how much water to drink during those times, consult your doctor, but a good rule of thumb for healthy people is two to three cups every hour or more if you're sweating significantly.

The following are some of the reasons why our bodies require water:

1. **It acts as a lubricant for the joints.**
   Cartilage, which is present in joints and spinal disks, is around 80% water. Dehydration over time can impair the joints' shock-absorbing abilities, resulting in joint pain.
2. **It is responsible for the production of saliva and mucus.**
   Saliva contributes to the digestive process and keeps the lips, nose, and eyes moist. It eliminates friction and wears and tear. Additionally, drinking water keeps the mouth

clean. When substituted for sugared beverages, it can also help prevent tooth decay.

3. **It is responsible for oxygen delivery throughout the body.**

   Blood is more than 90% water, and it transports oxygen to various regions of the body.

4. **4. It improves the health and appearance of the skin.**

   When the skin is dehydrated, it becomes more susceptible to skin diseases and premature aging.

5. **It protects the brain, spinal cord, and other delicate structures.**

   Dehydration can affect the brain's structure and function. Additionally, it plays a role in the synthesis of hormones and neurotransmitters. As a result, prolonged dehydration can impair one's ability to think and reason.

6. **It maintains a healthy body temperature.**

   When the body heats up, water stored in the middle layers of the skin rises to the skin's surface as sweat. It cools the body as it evaporates within the realm of sport. Having a sufficient amount of water in the body may help alleviate the physical strain caused by heat stress during exercise. However, additional investigation into these impacts is necessary.

7. **It is necessary for the digestive system.**

   The bowel needs water to function correctly. Dehydration can result in digestive issues, constipation, and a stomach that is too acidic. As a result, the risk of heartburn and stomach ulcers increases.

8. **It eliminates bodily waste.**

   Water is required for the processes of sweating and urination, and waste elimination.

9. **It aids in blood pressure regulation.**

   A deficiency of water can lead the blood to grow thicker, increasing blood pressure.

10. **It is necessary for the airways.**

    When a person is dehydrated, the body restricts the airways to limit water loss. As a result, it can aggravate asthma and allergies.

11. **It facilitates the accessibility of minerals and nutrients.**

These dissolve in water, allowing them to reach many regions of the body.

12. **It protects the kidneys from injury.**

    The kidneys are responsible for fluid regulation throughout the body. Therefore, inadequate water intake might result in kidney stones and other complications.

13. **It enhances athletic performance.**

    According to some research, drinking more water may improve performance during rigorous activity. While additional study is needed to validate this, one review discovered that dehydration impairs performance during activities lasting more than 30 minutes.

14. **Loss of weight**

    Water can also assist in weight loss when substituted for sugary drinks and sodas. In addition, by producing a sense of fullness, "preloading" with water before meals can help reduce overeating.

15. **It decreases the likelihood of experiencing a hangover.**

When partying, alternating unsweetened soda water with ice and lemon with alcoholic beverages can help reduce alcohol overconsumption.

HOW MUCH FOOD DO WE NEED?

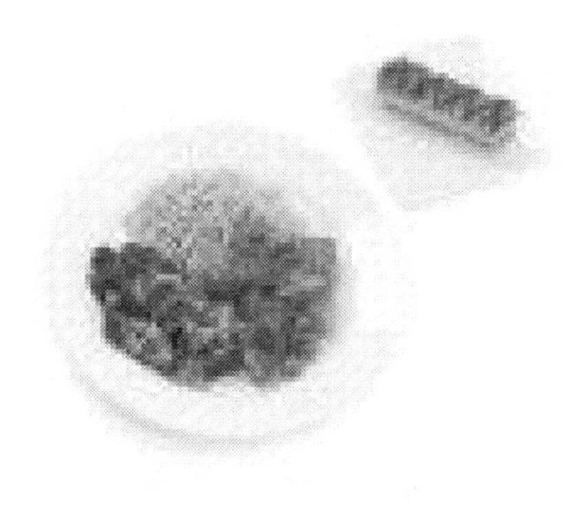

We are all aware—and you have already heard me deliver my registered dietitian monologue to lose weight, one must either consume less than one burns or burn more than one consumes. Identical distinction.

Depending on your personality type, this may sound more mathematically demanding than balancing a checkbook. And much worse if you're the type that never balances your checkbook.

The good news is that most of us will lose weight on a daily diet of 1,500 calories. (If you want to be even more specific with your calorie reduction, try this calculation to determine a daily calorie target that will help you lose a healthy 1 to 2 pounds per week.) OK, excellent, but what do 1,500 calories look like? It is the overall calorie count for everything seen here. Even better, here is a breakdown of the meals:

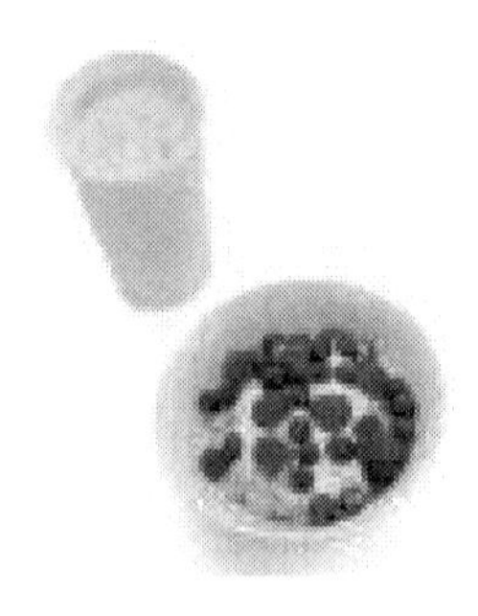

Breakfast: Consume 300–350 calories to kick-start your day. For instance, a 349-calorie breakfast here includes 1 cup of oats topped with 14 cups nonfat plain yogurt and 12 cup berries, as well as a 12 oz. Nonfat cappuccino.

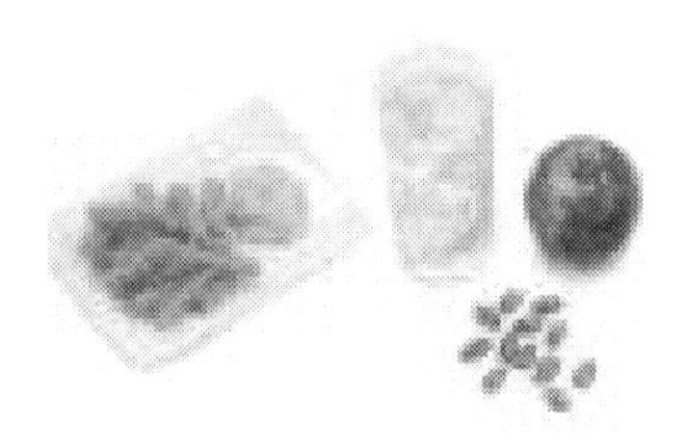

Snacks: Your daily snacks should contain between 250 and 375 calories, depending on how much you consume at meals. Two snacks are shown here, one for the morning and one for the afternoon. For example, a morning snack of 1 cup of baby carrots and 14 cups of hummus has a calorie count of 157. A snack of a tiny apple, 12 almonds, and ice water with lemon has 170 calories in the afternoon. Here are some additional snack alternatives for any time of day, all under 250 calories.

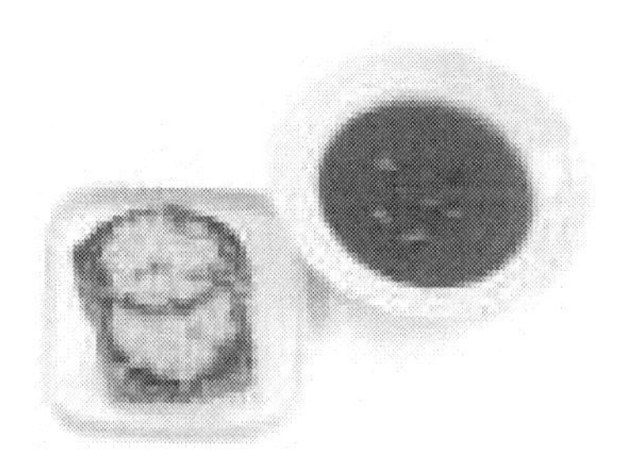

Lunch: Aim for 325–400 calories for lunch. What's pictured is 362 calories from one slice of whole-wheat bread toasted with 12 oz. Cheddar cheese and two tomato slices, as well as 112 cups of black bean soup. A little more portable alternative (for the workplace or a road trip, for example) is a tuna sandwich (2 pieces multigrain bread, 12 cup tuna salad made with two teaspoons low-fat mayonnaise, lettuce, tomato) and a peach (327 calories total).

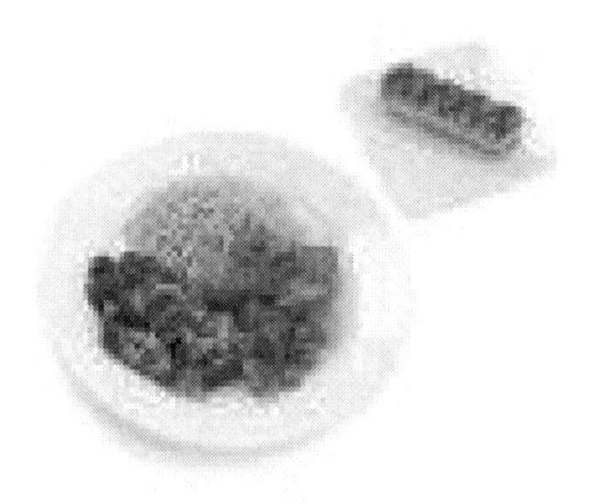

Dinner: Consume approximately 500 calories to round off your day. For instance, the illustrated Provencal Tuna Steaks with Sicilian-Style Broccoli, 12 cup pearl barley, and Baby Tiramisu for dessert contain only 481 calories.

Consider substituting dessert for a glass of wine with dinner. A 5-ounce glass of wine contains approximately 120 calories.

WHAT FUNCTION DO FATS PLAY IN HEALTH AND ENERGY PRODUCTION, AND WHAT ARE THEY?

The body uses fat as a fuel source, and fat is the body's primary energy storage medium. Fat serves a variety of additional functions in the body, and a moderate amount is required for overall health. Saturated, monounsaturated, and polyunsaturated fats are all types of fat found in food. Fats are the slowest source of energy, yet they are also the most energy-efficient. Fat provides the body with around nine calories per gram, more than twice as many proteins or carbohydrates. The body stores any surplus energy as fat because lipids are such an efficient type of energy. When a person acquires weight, pre-adipocytes in the connective tissue develop and fill with fat, forming adipocytes, storing fat as a possible energy source when food is scarce. Essential fatty acids, such as triglycerides, cholesterol, and other fatty acids that the body can't manufacture on its own, store energy, insulate us, and protect our key organs. They serve as messengers, assisting proteins in their functions. Fat also aids in absorbing fat-soluble vitamins such as A, D, E, and K. Fat also helps keep you warm by filling your fat cells and insulating your body. Your body acquires important fatty acids called linoleic and linolenic acids from the fats you eat. Adipose tissue can be found in the following places in humans: beneath the skin (subcutaneous fat), around internal organs (visceral fat), in bone marrow (yellow bone marrow), intermuscular (Muscular system), and the breast (breast tissue). Adipose tissue is located in adipose depots, which are specific places where adipose tissue can be found.

HOW CAN I PUT THE POWER PRESENT IN FOOD TO USE IN MY BODY?

All elements of the body (muscles, brain, heart, and liver) require energy to function. The food we eat provides this energy.

Our bodies mix the food we eat with fluids (acids and enzymes) in the stomach to digest it. When food is swallowed in the stomach, the carbohydrate content of the food (sugars and starches) is converted to glucose, a distinct type of sugar.

Before glucose is released into the bloodstream, it is absorbed in the stomach and small intestines. Our bodies, on the other hand, require insulin to utilize or store glucose for energy. Therefore, glucose lingers in the bloodstream without insulin, causing blood sugar levels to rise. At some time during the day, many people feel tired or rundown. A lack of energy can cause you to be less productive in your regular activities. Not surprisingly, the type and quantity of food you consume significantly impact your energy levels throughout the day.

Even though all foods provide energy, some foods provide nutrients that can help you maintain your energy levels and alertness, and attention throughout the day. Food is a storehouse of chemical energy. Chemical energy is stored in food as molecule bonds at the most fundamental level. Potential energy is represented by molecular bonds, which can be very stable, as in fat molecules, or very active and transient, as in ATP molecules.

Although oxygen-rich blood rushes through your body to your heart, muscles, and brain anytime you exercise, it is a natural energy enhancer for accessing and containing the power of food. Fitting a workout into your day regularly, even if it's only for 10 minutes at a time, will help you maintain your energy levels. Through the food chain, energy is exchanged between creatures. For example, photosynthesis is how plants get their energy from the sun. This energy can then be transmitted down the food chain from one organism to the next. The producer is the organism that derives energy from sunshine. It is yet another method of gaining access to the food's power.

Means of accessing food power

1. Fill a boiling tube with cold water.
2. Take note of the water's initial temperature.
3. Tally the weight of the food sample.
4. Cook the stuff over high heat until it catches fire.
5. Use the flame from the burning food to heat the water.
6. Take note of the water's final temperature.

HOW TO SPEND LESS TIME ON MONEY AND FOOD

Purchasing food these days can be a real hassle. It's critical to budget carefully so that you don't spend your entire income on groceries. The difficult thing is knowing how to spend sensibly while not forsaking necessities. You can set yourself on the right track to eating well on a budget by following these 15 steps. If you spend ten minutes watching the news or going through Facebook, you'll quickly understand how much is beyond your control. You'll see proof of greed, corruption, natural disasters, and sickness in just ten minutes. Even the most composed of us can feel overwhelmed. Although you have no control over the new, there is one thing you do have control over that is far more powerful. You'll have the energy you need to deal with life's daily stresses if you choose to eat wisely. Furthermore, eating healthy has been proved to promote immunity, lower blood pressure, and mental wellness, among other things.

I'm sure this isn't the first time you've heard about the numerous advantages of eating well. A fast search on Google yields 1.7 billion results. The information is readily available and unrestricted. But, unfortunately, fewer than 10% of adults and adolescents in the United States consume enough fruits and vegetables. So let's look at why we have trouble eating healthy and how we may remedy it.

1. Don't Make Impulsive Purchases

What I mean is that when you go shopping for groceries, focus solely on what you require rather than on what appears to be appealing. It's quite easy to go into a supermarket for a gallon of milk and leave with $30 worth of junk food that you don't need but bought because it looked delicious.

2. Go to the store with your blinders on.

When shopping for food, it can be somewhat distracting. Always avoid purchasing something if you are unsure whether or not it will be used. If you're going to the grocery store to buy milk, bread, or eggs, head right to those sections and then check out.

3. Purchase Frozen Foods

It is an excellent idea for canned and dry products as well. In my family, we buy these goods in bulk when they are cheaper and save money in the long term when the price rises. However, you have to worry about perishable commodities more frequently because they have a long supply life.

4. Take your lunches with you

It is the one that always catches people's attention. It's just easier to stop at a fast-food place or eat from a vending machine these days than it is to pack a lunch. The disadvantage is that you are risking your health and your finances by overspending on food that isn't worth it. You can spend $5 on a burger and fries or half that amount on packed lunch and get twice as much food.

5. Make the Most of Your Leftovers

Now, I'm not sure about you, but virtually every time we cook dinner in my house, we always end up with leftovers. Simply repurposing these leftovers is a great strategy to reduce food waste and save money. So, if you're anything like me, you'll take these leftovers to work with you. With just one stone, you can kill two birds.

6. Restaurant Meals Should Be Shared

It is one step that I wish I had known about earlier. If you share meals when you go out to eat, you may save a lot of money while still having a wonderful time. If you think about it, you nearly always have a lot of leftover food at the end of your meals, so why not pick something you and someone else both like and divide it?

7. Download a Grocery App

In your effort to save money, using a shopping app might be beneficial. For example, you may use it to look at the store's deals while you're there, to look for exclusive offers (if you're a member), and to keep track of what you're buying and spending.

8. Make a family shopping list that everyone can see.

If you live in a fast-paced, always-on-the-go family, this will come in handy. Everyone can contribute to a cooperative shopping list kept in the house, making it easy for whoever does the shopping. Another advantage is that it helps cut down on unnecessary grocery purchases that might otherwise go to waste.

9. Establish Weekly Goals

It is unquestionable one of the most basic notions, but it is also one of the most difficult to grasp, yet it is achievable! You can easily keep track of your expenditures by setting a weekly spending limit.

10. Don't Be Afraid to Shop Off-Brand

There's no guilt in buying off-brand or store-brand merchandise. These are almost always less expensive than name-brand things, and you can't tell the difference most of the time.

11. Take advantage of the sales

Always look for sales in your local newspaper. Why not take advantage of the fact that you may always find good prices while buying this way? Additionally, you may save money by deciding which grocery store to visit based on the greatest prices.

12. Learn how to use coupons.

We've all seen those extreme couponers on TV, the ones who go to great lengths to clip coupons to save money. So why not join this group of people? Of course, you don't have to go to extremes like the people on TV to save money on groceries, but clipping coupons can help you save money.

13. Join us as a member

Many companies offer free small memberships that require you to pick up a rewards card, sign up by email, and start saving. In addition, you may be eligible for special discounts and coupons, and some retailers will reward you with points toward merchandise. These perks can help you save money on groceries and even earn money off of gas in some cases.

14. Choose from the Value Menu

Eating from the value menu is another method to save money when dining out. When you eat out this way, you may obtain enough food to fill you up for a fraction of the price. This way, you can still enjoy eating out without having to spend full price.

15. Set a Boundary

One of the most effective budgeting strategies is to take the amount of money you have available to spend on food each month and withdraw it in cash. After that, split the money into four envelopes and label them with the weeks (week #1, week #2, and so on). Then, each week, only use one envelope and spend only what's in it.

Spending money on meals can be more stressful than it has to be, so why not attempt to make it as painless as possible? I hope these suggestions are as useful to you as they have been to me.

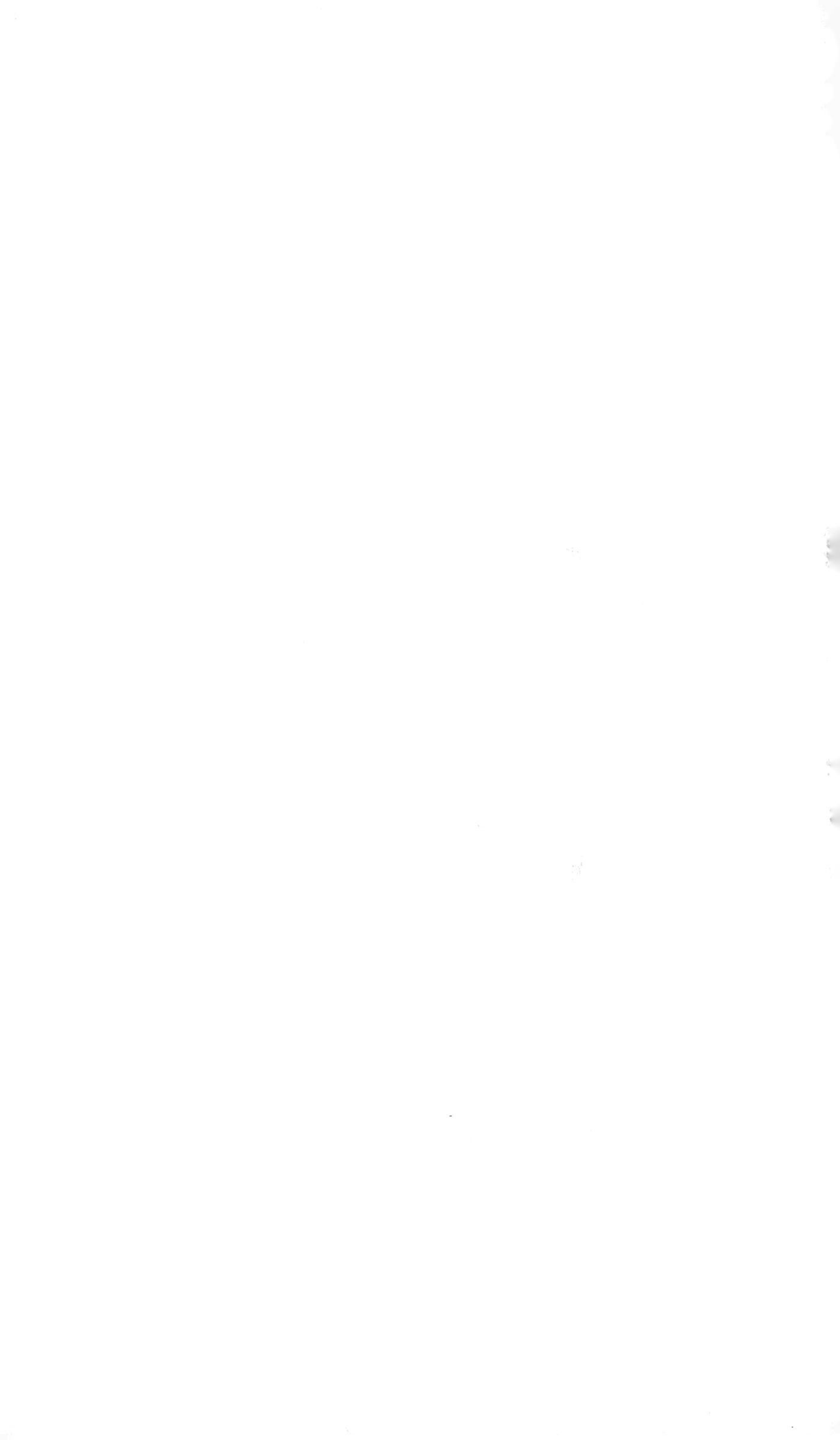